Christiane Voßemer

# "I want to be somewhere!"

# Perspectives on Development

edited by

Petra Dannecker
(Universität Wien)

and

Ulrike Schultz
(Theologische Hochschule Friedensau)

Volume 2

LIT

Christiane Voßemer

# "I want to be somewhere!"

## Young Malawian Nurses' Perspectives on Migration

LIT

Cover image: Katharina Voßemer, 2018

**Bibliographic information published by the Deutsche Nationalbibliothek**
The Deutsche Nationalbibliothek lists this publication in the Deutsche Nationalbibliografie; detailed bibliographic data are available on the Internet at http://dnb.d-nb.de.

ISBN 978-3-643-90872-8 (pb)
ISBN 978-3-643-95872-3 (PDF)

**A catalogue record for this book is available from the British Library.**


Klosbachstr. 107
CH-8032 Zürich
Tel. +41 (0) 44-251 75 05
E-Mail: zuerich@lit-verlag.ch http://www.lit-verlag.ch
**Distribution:**
In the UK: Global Book Marketing, e-mail: mo@centralbooks.com
In North America: Independent Publishers Group, e-mail: orders@ipgbook.com
In Germany: LIT Verlag Fresnostr. 2, D-48159 Münster
Tel. +49 (0) 2 51-620 32 22, Fax +49 (0) 2 51-922 60 99, e-mail: vertrieb@lit-verlag.de
e-books are available at www.litwebshop.de

# "I want to be somewhere!"

*Young Malawian Nurses' Perspectives on Migration*

*Christiane Voßemer, Vienna and Hamburg*

# TABLE OF CONTENTS

# *Lists of Figures, Tables and Pictures*

## *Figures*



## *Tables*



## *Annex Tables*



## *Pictures*

## *Preface*

This book provides a unique und compelling analysis of health migration from Malawi. An issue, which is, given the ways in which migration is currently discussed and 'managed', extremely valid. This especially since Christiane Voßemer rather than simply studying the reasons why people migrate, weaves the narratives of students who are aiming to achieve a nursing degree with conceptual reflections about the global context of health worker's international migration. In particular the analysis how this context gets reflected in the future visions and the life planning of the mainly female students is extremely innovative.

This focus on the life course visions of migration in the next generation of Malawian nurses draws attention to the social images about migration and their entanglement with gender and development in this part of the world. Images which are framing and influencing, as shown, not only the future professional life projects of the students but are shaping concepts and ideas of partnership, families, personal developments, and social and economic status, dimensions which are silenced in mainstream migration research.

It is especially the author's actor-oriented approach, namely placing nursing students in Malawi at the center, which provides the reader with insights into international health migration and explanations for the health crisis in the Global South. A crisis closely related to migration policies in the Global North, especially the competition for skilled migrants in general and skilled workers for the heath sector in particular. The biographies of the students offer a means to go beyond simplistic and purely economic reasoning why people move.

The insightful analysis and the discussions Christiane Voßemer presents in her book are not only a valuable contribution to migration and development studies but also policy makers. On one hand, policy makers in countries facing outmigration and brain drain of skilled workers in the health sector and beyond are provided with a discussion of different coping strategies. On the other hand, and given the current academic and political discussion in the Global North, this publication should be read as a reminder that the current migration situation is the result of a history of persisting unequal power relations and policies between the Global South and the Global North.

*Petra Dannecker*

## *Abstract*

Malawi's shortage of human resources for health has been a major concern of the country's Ministry of Health and its development partners throughout the past decades. One dimension of the crisis, the international migration of nurses, is the focus of this book. It tackles in particular future nurse migration as it explores biographic aspects of migration intentions among young nursing graduates, guided by the following study questions: How far are migration intentions relevant to the life planning of students with a degree in nursing? Which collective experiences and ideas of migration, which life scripts and self-identities explain this relevance? Which consequences arise from these findings for policies to improve the retention of nurses in the Malawian health system and the gains from nurses' migration respectively?

Guided by a micro-sociological approach to migration and life planning, this exploratory study is based in empirical data collected using qualitative research methods and analysed using the Grounded Theory methodology (Glaser and Strauss 2005). It traces and clarifies the biographic anchors of young nursing graduates' migration intentions in their professional, personal, partnership and family-related, socio-economic and religiously guided life projects. In each realm, interactions between young nurses' migration intentions and biographically guiding concepts of life, cultures of migration and self-identities are traced.

The young nursing graduates' narratives of migration and successful return reflect a (post)colonial symbolic capital of migration, globalized self-identities as well as ethical bonds of family solidarity and reciprocity. Their migration prospects are mostly framed as migration-to-study projects and insert into their life plans as an essential *rite of passage*, connected with ideas of professional career, gender empowerment, individualization, modern lifestyles and membership to a global as well as local elite. The desires to migrate are grounded in self-identities that emphasize personal entitlements to make individual choices, pursue ambitious life plans and access globally available resources. By contrast, the state of the Malawian health system and the working conditions of nurses in particular, as well as local constellations of gendered social roles are perceived as fundamental barriers to realize individual professional and private life projects. This disparity establishes a high migration potential among young nursing graduates.

Nevertheless, also prospects for the nurses' future return to, respectively their later retention in the Malawian health system become tangible: they express a strong sense of affiliation to nursing for women, to the health sector for men nurses, an appreciation for continuous training opportunities in the public system, and positive ideas about a future life in Malawi. Based on the gained biographic insights, the last chapter gives suggestions regarding policies to promote successful temporary migration and return mobility. These concern the political recognition of the persistent migration potential, the strengthening of informed migration decision-making, improved access to postgraduate studies, the active management of interational migration, the promotion of engagement from abroad, and the opening of return perspectives, including ways to make the profession in Malawi more attractive to young nurses' eyes.

## *Acknowledgements*

As a young researcher, conducting this research and writing this book were challenging and compelling experiences. I was lucky to count on the support of many inspiring people, I would like to thank here. I cannot miss the opportunity to express my sincere gratitude and appreciation in the first place to every nursing student participating in a research workshop or even giving me her or his time for a personal interview, despite the packed and stressful everyday life of a student in times of writing final research reports and preparing graduation exams. Thank you for allowing me to learn from you and for the dense and valuable experience of getting to know your lives and thoughts! Your interest and commitment to take part in this study made the data collection the greatest pleasure for me.

Different supervisors and mentors advised me during my stay in Malawi and in the aftermath, helped me to get to know my field of research, counselled me in managing formal procedures and the process of writing-up my work. I am very grateful for this support and know well that this work would not have been successful without you. In particular, I wish to acknowledge the perseverant guidance from Univ. Prof. Dr. Petra Dannecker, my supervisor at University of Vienna, the counselling of Juliane Ilse (GTZ Malawi German Health Programme), whose feedback and encouragement guided me through the data collection and first drafting process, and the helpful and patient advice from my local supervisor, Andrew Simwaka from Kamuzu College of Nursing.

I thank all lecturers and officials in Malawi who offered me their time and assistance and allowed me insight into their experiences and registers, as well as to the team of GTZ, offering their helping hands wherever needed. The information of Maureen Shirwa and Anni Msosa from UNIMA/KCN, Veronica Maluwa and Chrissie Chilomba from NMCM, and Harriet Kapyepye from NONM have been of essential help to improve my background understanding and open the field for this research.

Furthermore, I feel indebted to my friend Anna Sophia Schultz for her very helpful, conscientious and rigorous feedback on my work. Caroline Matululu corrected many pages of transcripts with great commitment, and Marianne Kupper made herself available for several overnight language checks. Last but not least, the love, generosity and patience of Dietmar and my daughters accompanied me throughout the always-stretching time of finalizing this book.

Christiane Voßemer
Hamburg, August 2018

## *Abbreviations*

| | |
|---|---|
| BSc | Bachelor of Science |
| DFID | UK Department for International Development |
| DHO/DNO | District Health Office(r) / District Nursing Office(r) |
| EHRP | Emergency Human Resources (for Health) Programme |
| GCP | Global Code of Practice for the Recruitment of Health Workers |
| GDC / GIZ (GTZ) | German Development Cooperation / German Organisation for International Co-operation (till 2011 German Organisation for Technical Co-operation) |
| GoM | Government of Malawi |
| HR(H) | Human Resources (for Health) |
| ILO | International Labour Organisation |
| IMG | International Medical Graduates |
| InWEnt | Capacity Building International, since 2011 part of GIZ |
| IOs | International Organisations |
| JLI | Joint Learning Initiative on Human Resources for Health |
| KCN | Kamuzu College of Nursing |
| MCM | Medical Council of Malawi |
| MDGs | Millennium Development Goals |
| MDHS | Malawi Demographic and Health Survey |
| MoH | Ministry of Health Malawi |
| MoL/SoL | Ministry of Labour Malawi / Secretary of Labour Malawi |
| MSc | Master of Science |
| MSCE | Malawi School Certificate of Education |
| NHS | National Health Service of the United Kingdom |
| NGO | Non-governmental Organisation |
| NMCM | Nurses and Midwives Council of Malawi |
| NONM | National Organisation of Nurses and Midwifes Malawi |

| | |
|---|---|
| NORAD | Norwegian Agency for Development Co-operation |
| OECD | Organisation for Economic Co-operation and Development |
| PHD | Doctorate of Philosophy |
| RoM | Republic of Malawi |
| SADC | Southern African Development Community |
| SWAp | Sector Wide Approach (of Development Co-operation) |
| UK NMC | United Kingdom Nurses and Midwives Council |
| UNIMA | University of Malawi |
| UN-DESA | United Nations Department of Economic and Social Affairs |
| UNFPA | United Nations Population Fund |
| UNICEF | United Nations Children's Fund |
| VSO | Volunteer Services International |
| WHA/WHO | World Health Assembly / World Health Organisation |
| ZAR | Republic of South Africa |

# I. INTRODUCTION

International migration of nurses from Malawi constitutes one important factor in the country's severe human resources for health crisis. As is adumbrated in the book title "*I want to be somewhere*" (the statement of a young nurse I interviewed) the longing for a move abroad still guides many young nurses' life plans substantially. This book deals with their intentions and images of international migration[1] and aims to strengthen the often-neglected biographical perspective in research and policy development on international migration of nurses from the *Global South*.

The study focuses on life course visions of migration in the next generation of Malawian degree nurses. Diverse biographic aspects of their migration intentions are explored guided by the following study questions: How far are migration intentions relevant to the life planning of students with a degree in nursing? Which collective experiences and ideas of migration, which life scripts and self-identities explain this relevance? How can the findings inform (development) policies to improve the retention of nurses in the Malawian health system and the brain gain from nurses' migration? Throughout the analysis, the biographic anchors of young nursing graduates' migration intentions are traced, considering their concepts of life and self-identities, as well as social images of migration.

The book falls into 5 parts. Following this introduction, *part two* describes the background of the study, sketching out the global context of heath workers' international migration from developing to developed countries and detailing main patterns of nurse migration that have emerged from previous research on (in particular African) health workers' migration intentions. In a third step, the Malawian context of nurse migration is introduced, describing

---

[1] Unless otherwise specified, *migration* in this book always refers to international labour and student migration.

quantitative trends as well as qualitative patterns of Malawian nurses' international migration and the country's human resources for health challenges and policy interventions.

*Part three* provides an outline of the research project, presenting the research design, central concepts and approaches drawn upon and the methods as well as limitations of data collection and analysis. Taking a micro-sociological approach to migration and life planning, empirical data was collected on behalf of an exploratory research design using qualitative research methods. A combination of group discussions and in-depth interviews allowed to inquire into the interwoven concepts of life and migration in the students' biographic and career choices as well as their life planning, offering profound insights into biographical dimensions of migration recurrent in this group of young nurses. The grounded theory methodology (Glaser and Strauss 2005) served to structure the research process and analyse the data.

*Part four* discusses the research findings on students' visions of migration and is organized along different areas of their life plans. Introductory, an overview about main characteristics of their life plans is given, highlighting relevant self-identities and scripts of life, as well as identifying six central *biographical horizons*. Migration is found to constitute an essential element of most students' life plans, connected with ideas of professional career, gender empowerment, individualization and modern lifestyles that insert migration into their overall biographic perspective as a *rite of passage* to obtain an elite position in the Malawian society. The graduates' biographic migration projects are grounded in self-identities that emphasize the personal entitlement to make individual choices, pursue ambitious life plans and access globally available resources. By contrast, the current conditions of the Malawian health system, the working conditions of nurses as well as constellations of social roles are perceived as fundamental barriers to realize the individual professional and private life plan.

At the same time the students' narratives of migration and successful return reflect the (post)colonial symbolic capital of migration, personal membership aspirations to global and local communities of privilege as well as ethical bonds of family solidarity and reciprocity. The sub-chapters of part four analyse the nurses' biographic reasoning about and function of migration prospects in the six *biographical horizons* identified: particular emphasis is given to the ***professional life project***, which centres concerns about educational and professional career advancement, the status of the nursing profession, discrimination related to gender and age, as well as the working conditions for bedside nurses. The nurses' biographic projects related to ***partnership and parenthood***, respectively single life, shape distinctive, gendered migration projects, accommodating the needs of the couple and social concern regarding marriage and personal independence. ***Family bonds*** of obligations and support establish a tangible influence of extended families of origin on the young graduates' future plans. Their interests are built into the personal migration projects in ways that promise to allow negotiating and balancing responsibilities and personal ambitions. Migration is sought as a biographic *rite of passage* also in the realm of ***personal development***, where the students associate migration with the exposure to modern lifestyles, personal independence and membership to a mobile global academic elite. Adopting ***religious guidance*** by a Christian God as fundamental to any life and future decisions, religious ideas and practices are either subtly or explicitly considered within the migration projects as well. Last but not least, the young nurses' migration projects are heavily charged with expectations to translate academic achievements into elite ***social and socioeconomic status*** within the Malawian context. Their ambitions intimately link to ideas of making social contributions in the home society, mirroring common discourses of a migration and development mantra.

*Part five* condenses the previous discussions with a view to address political consequences that may be derived from the study findings. It takes a meta-perspective on the analysis to point out the central biographic dimensions of young nursing graduates' migration intentions. Based on this, the biographic potentials of their migration from, return to, and retention in the Malawian health care system are elaborated. While pointing to a high migration potential in the young generation of highly qualified nurses, also potentials for their retention in, respectively their return to the Malawian health system are identified: a strong sense of affiliation to nursing and the health sector, an appreciation for the continuous training opportunities available and positive ideas about a future life in Malawi. Policy makers are alerted to different problem areas meriting political attention in order to cope with the perpetual migration potential. Namely, it is suggested to recognize the migration potential politically, strengthen informed migration decision-making, build better access to postgraduate studies, revisit international approaches to restrict mobility critically, negotiate international migration agreements, promote engagement from abroad as well as the opening of return prospects, and last but importantly intensify the efforts to make working in the nursing profession in Malawi more attractive. Concluding this book, I mention contributions of the study findings to the literature on migration of nurses in Malawi and beyond and look towards areas of further study interest.

# II. MALAWIAN NURSE MIGRATION IN CONTEXT

## Global Nurse Migration

### *A Looming Global Health Workforce Crisis*

"There is a global shortage of health workers, with some of the most serious shortfalls occurring in sub-Saharan Africa, where the situation reflects the devastating impact of HIV/AIDS on health workers, accelerating labour migration and the legacy of underinvestment in human resources." (Mangham 2007: 1)

As health care delivery is by nature a labour-intensive field, in particular in resource scare settings, the supply with human resources for health constitutes a critical input for the performance of health systems in developing countries (ibid.). This human resource supply is currently facing a systematic and global crisis in which already existing shortages are projected to severe, following a global trend of increasing demand and decreasing availability (OECD 2008; JLI 2004).

The Joint Learning Initiative on Human Resources for Health (JLI) outlined three major reasons: a neglect towards investment needs for human resources for health, the emergence of a global market for most cadres of health workers and the HIV/AIDS crisis (ibid.). The second and third reason hit poor countries in Sub-Sahara Africa particularly hard: austerity politics in the face of the financial and socioeconomic crisis have shaped health system reforms in many African countries since the 1980^s^, leading to a lack of resources to finance staff and offer adequate working conditions and, as a consequence, reducing the countries' competitiveness on the global market of health workers in terms of the offered working and living conditions. An increasing burden of disease, in particular but not solely resulting from the spread of the HIV/AIDS epidemic since the 1990^s^, has severed the working conditions of African health personnel on the ground. These conditions and lacking resources and capacities to recruit, train, manage and retain their workforce have driven the health systems of vulnerable countries like Malawi into a serious health worker shortage. (Omaswa 2009)

At the same time the demand for foreign health workers in OECD countries has been increasing due to a mismatch between investment into the training and retention of domestic health workers as well as demographic developments (OECD 2008). In order to meet this demand or temporarily fill the gaps, several OECD countries like the UK and the USA have been relying increasingly on international health workers, in particular nurses and physicians from overseas countries (ibid.; Pond and McPake 2006). Active, often aggressive recruitment practices have attracted an alarming share of the nursing workforce from Sub-Sahara African countries with serious shortages of health workers to "move west" (Mills 2008).

While those dynamics reflect how migration of the health workforce inscribes into the current conditions of health systems worldwide, a broader perspective on the phenomenon opens with when considering the historical and colonial context of health workers' migration on the one hand, an increasing mobility of highly skilled professionals in the context of globalisation on the other hand.

### *Nurse Migration: A Historic Phenomenon*

International migration of health workers is an old and cross-regional phenomenon that has become a global matter throughout the last two decades, when its patterns have seen considerable changes. Already in 1948, with the establishment of the UK National Health Service, local selection committees for the recruitment of nurses and midwives were founded in many British colonies in Africa (Likupe 2005). For countries like the Philippines but also India large-scale outmigration of doctors and nurses was common in the 1970s already (Bach 2003). The sending of Filipinas to the USA to be trained as nurses started in 1911, only one decade after the United States' take-over of the island. The sending of American women to the Philippines to train native women soon replaced this migration, but the high unemployment of Filipina nurses in the scarcely funded local health care system encouraged a renewed trend of Filipina nurses' migration to the USA that has continued as a gendered and racialized pattern of migration into the postcolonial times. (Schultheiss 2010; Ball 2004)

Today the Philippines are the major source country of international nurses, and the migration of Filipina nurses is encouraged politically as a means to fight unemployment and raise the national income in remittances. The substantial contribution of overseas nurses to their home countries' national income has even led to an economic dependence on their steady "export" and to the formulation of regional policies and bilateral agreements with major destination countries. The Philippines today give an example of a country actively managing migration, promoting outmigration of health workers and international agreements with receiving countries. Beyond economic benefits and dependencies, the migration of Nurses from the Philippines as from other countries in the *Global South* also generates major challenges - for the domestic health sector and society and for migrants' rights alike. (Ibid.)

First concerns about a medical *brain drain* date back as early as the 1950^s^ and 60^s^, when the extension of welfare states led to a first wave of immigration of doctors (and to a lower extend nurses) in particular to Australia, Canada, Germany, the UK and the USA (Bach 2003). The term *brain drain* reflects the idea that the migration of skilled professionals necessarily implies an economic and social loss to their country of origin. *Brain gain* in turn is referred to, when benefits of skilled migration to the country of origin are in focus, created e.g. via remittances and international social and business network or, in the case of circular migration and return, higher qualified and international professional experience enriching the local workforce.

In many countries of the *Global South*[1] the colonizers had introduced modern nursing and South-North migration of health

[1] In the context of the age of globalization, the terms *Global South* and *Global North* have increasingly been replacing the Cold War concept of a *First, Second*

workers has traditionally targeted prominently the respective countries of colonization (Alonso-Garbayo and Maben 2009; Raghuram 2009). Beyond such colonial linkages, patterns of international nurse migration had long taken the shape of South-South or North-North migration respectively, while South-North mobility among nurses, as well as the migration of other mid-level health cadres, only gained significance in recent years (Kingma 2007). Since the late 1990s the phenomenon of relatively large-scale health worker migration has furthermore extended to countries that had seemed to be fairly immune against it in the past. Those countries, several of which are located in Sub-Saharan Africa, have since been drawn into the dynamics of an increasingly integrated global labour market, to which migration had become a "significant and volatile component of human resource planning" (Bach 2003).

### *Health Workers in the 'Brain Drain' Debate*

Today, nurses' migration is part of the global labour mobility among highly qualified professionals in general (Zlotnik 2003). While women nurses represent a considerable share in the migration of qualified women, nurse migration reflects wider dynamics of migration among health workers and the highly skilled more generally quite closely.

> "Comparing the share of foreign-born doctors or nurses to the share of foreign-born in professional occupations or PhD holders shows that migrant health professionals are generally not overrepresented (see Dumont and Zurn, 2007). The higher the percentage of foreign-born among highly-skilled workers is, the higher it is also for doctors and nurses." (OECD 2008: 30)

In a national health system perspective as well as in migration studies, the migration of health workers is perceived as an urgent politi-

---

and *Third World*. The term *Global South* signifies the position of formerly colonized states in the current world order, not on the world map. Different to the term *developing countries*, it is to be regarded as a momentum concept for a new international order reversing the subordinate position of formerly colonized countries. (Grovogui 2010) cal and economical problem. Within the development policy discussion, the migration of highly qualified medical professionals has become the prime example for *brain drain*, i.e. the conceptual approach towards mobility of the highly qualified that highlights the losses and negative consequences on developing source countries. Those tend to be more tangible and non-tradable in the labour and skill intensive health system than in other areas of the economy (Vinokur 2006; Skeldon 2005). At the same time, it is regarded as a general pattern of (in particular early) migration flows that they are selective to the highly skilled and educated. The migration of the most educated to national and international centres is seen as a factor that increases the unequal relations and productivities between peripheral and central regions within a country as well as internationally, as has been argued by the world-system-theory of migration (Massey et al. 1993).

At the same time the concept of *brain drain* as well as the question whether international migration of the highly-skilled is to be regarded as a loss or a gain to a developing source country have been discussed critically and controversially under economic, sociological as well as political development perspectives (Skeldon 2005). One body of studies calls into question that health workers' migration has a negative impact on health indicators and points to positive effects on domestic educational investment (Bhargava, Docquier and Moullan 2011; Docquier and Rapoport 2011). Secondly, the methodologically individualist and nationalist approaches guiding the *brain drain* debate have been jeopardized, arguing that the concept reduces the multidirectional mobility, activity and relatedness of highly-skilled migrants to the question whether an individual stood in the borders of a nation or not, thereby neglecting the global systemic dimensions of the phenomenon (Vinokur 2006; Skeldon 2005). Thirdly and related to the previous points, the debate has put forward two different concepts: *brain gain*, accounting for the potential of qualified migrants to generate positive effects on development in the country they left –

as *diaspora* members[2], agents in transnational networks or skilled temporary returnees (ibid.), and *brain circulation*, highlighting the persistent mobility of the highly-skilled between different destinations, including their home country, that may create an international pool of human talents to the benefit of all source and destination countries (Tung 2008).

Those new concepts have likewise attracted criticism from different angles. It has been pointed out that *brain gain* effects do not emerge automatically, but depend on political conditions. According to findings of Docquier and Rapoport (2011) from a broad review of economic studies, source countries can generate gains from migration of the highly skilled. However, losses and gains from migration depend fundamentally on source countries' public policies and abilities "to capitalize on the incentives for human capital formation in a context of migration and seize the global benefits from having a skilled, educated diaspora" (ibid. 51).
Other critics doubt whether in the case of *medical migration*[3] these dynamics could gain the same strength and benefits as e.g. in the context of IT-professionals (Skeldon 2005; Vinokur 2006). Contrariwise, some authors point to the necessity to capture medical migration as part of a modern phenomenon of *brain circulation* among the highly skilled, and to recognize the existing contributions of active medical diasporas (ibid.; IOM 2007; for Malawi: Grigulis 2010; Lwanda 2007).

The new acknowledgement of the *brain gain* potential of migration reflects a paradigmatic change of the political and scientific approach towards migration and its impact on development, described by Faist and Reisenauer as a "migration-development mantra" (2009: 2). The authors argue that the scientific discourse

---

[2] In migration studies the term *diaspora* is commonly referred to when talking about clearly or loosely subscribed groups of migrants who relate to or engage with their home country, e.g. funding institutions, opening businesses or social organisations, making investments or engaging in political processes.

[3] The debate on *medical migration* is focused on physicians and medical specialist. However, as the nurses approached in this study are trained academically at length and hold internationally recognized qualifications, they are to be considered relevant to the debate as well.

on the *migration-development nexus* has been reshaped in recent years by a new political discourse that establishes a *migration-development mantra*, conceptualizing migration as a solution, rather than a problem of development. From a discourse analytical perspective, the authors warn that this new mantra may not be credited as a new scientific ground to describe the nexus of migration and development. Rather it should be analysed as a reflection of societal discourses and political interests in the Global North to emphasize that migrations of the highly skilled would enhance developing countries' profit.

The general contextualization of nurse migration in this subchapter points to the close linkages local health systems with global health markets and overall migration trends especially among the highly skilled in creating medical migration as a global phenomenon. The international migration of nurses holds strong traditions and a particular history of gendered colonial relations that can be of importance in approaching nurses prospects of migration in present days as well.

### Factors and Patterns of Nurse Migration

„If something is in abundance, it is reasons to move." (Arango 2000: 293)

From a national health system perspective, four interacting, encouraging or inhibiting factors have been identified for the migration of health workers: the attractiveness of source and recipient institutions and countries, their respective training capacities, social, financial or legal borders to migrate and attrition due to reasons other than migration. (Padarath et al. 2003)

Dynamics of international migration add to the internal mobility of health workers from rural to urban areas as well as from public to private health systems, which are mayor concerns for the health systems of Southern African countries and beyond. International migration requires higher resource inputs and therefore tends to be associated with stronger *push* and/or *pull* factors than internal mobility.[4] Both often follow similar educational, occupational and economic drives, amended in the case of international migration by prospects related to the different environment associated with a move abroad.

From the conducted literature review a broad variety of factors, dynamics and concepts of nurse migration evolved, building a frame of reference and embedding for the individual migrations intentions focused in this study, and allowing a contextualization and discussion of the empirical findings with regard to the global perspective on the migration of nurses. Based on a literature review on international migration of African health workers in general and nurses in particular. Table 1 (next page) gives a compilation of the wider spectrum of exogenous and endogenous factors relevant for nurses' motivations to migrate based on Padarath et al. 2004; VSO 2010; van Eyck 2004; Alonso-Garbayo and Maben 2009; Dovlo 2003.

Health workers' individual reasons to migrate tend to go beyond the spectrum of professional factors focused under a national health system perspective, as Figure 1 shows.

Beyond the multitude of structural factors at stake, it should be kept in mind that the *interaction between different variables* as well as their s*ocial and individual connotation* seem to be of foremost importance in understanding why and how migration takes place. Studies on nurses' intentions to migrate reveal e.g. an ambivalent role of family, personal and social aspects in decisions to move (Larsen et al. 2005; Grigulis 2010). General literature on migration, in particular on the migration of women and of health workers, as well as specific literature on nurse migration from different countries in the *Global South* informs on several relational categories, bridging and underlying different factors.[5]

---

[4] In migration studies, conditions urging people to leave a country (e.g. low income or unemployment) are referred to as *push factors*. attractive conditons in destination countries (e.g. higher standard of living or better access to education) are called *pull factors*. Unless otherwise specified, *migration* in this book always refers to international labour and student migration.

[5] I draw these points mainly from a literature review on nurse migration from different African source countries to the UK, but include also general literature on health workers' migration.

*Table 1. Factors Encouraging/ Inhibiting Nurse Migration*

| | | |
|---|---|---|
| ENCOURAGING MIGRATION | **PUSH factors** | **Exogenous to the health system:**<br>low, insecure quality of life, lack of educational opportunities, crime, war, conflict, repression<br>**Endogenous to the health system:**<br>low remuneration, social security and pension benefits, lack of job satisfaction, work associated risks<br>health system governance/ occupational environment (bureaucracy, inefficiency)<br>lack of satisfactory further education and career development opportunities |
| | **PULL factors** | **Exogenous:**<br>Quality of life and lifestyle, education for children, freedom of speech<br>**Endogenous:**<br>Higher remuneration, social security and pension benefits, centralisation of health institutions<br>Health system governance/occupational environment (promotion opportunities, efficiency)<br>More satisfying & safer working conditions, quality of advanced health institutions<br>Educational and career development opportunities, international recruitment |
| | **MOVE ON factors** | Transnational communities and networks<br>Entrance requirements of the envisaged final destination<br>Encouraging/inhibiting dynamics between the first and the following recipient countries |
| INHIBITING MIGRATION | **RETAIN factors** | Levels of morale, success and social recognition, rewards and incentives<br>Family kinship, social and cultural ties, patriotism |
| | **REPEL factors** | Immigration procedures, language- and cultural barriers, xenophobia and discrimination<br>Different clinical practices |
| | **STAY factors** | New social and cultural bonds, disrupt of new lifestyle patterns, interruption of education of children<br>Ignorance of job opportunities in the source country<br>Citizenship requirements in destination countries, non-transferability of social security benefits |
| | **BAR-RIERS** | Immigration and visa restrictions, recruitment bans e.g. by Codes of Practice<br>Financial costs of migration |

*Figure 1. Health Workers' Reasons to Migrate in Cameroon, South Africa, Uganda and Zimbabwe*

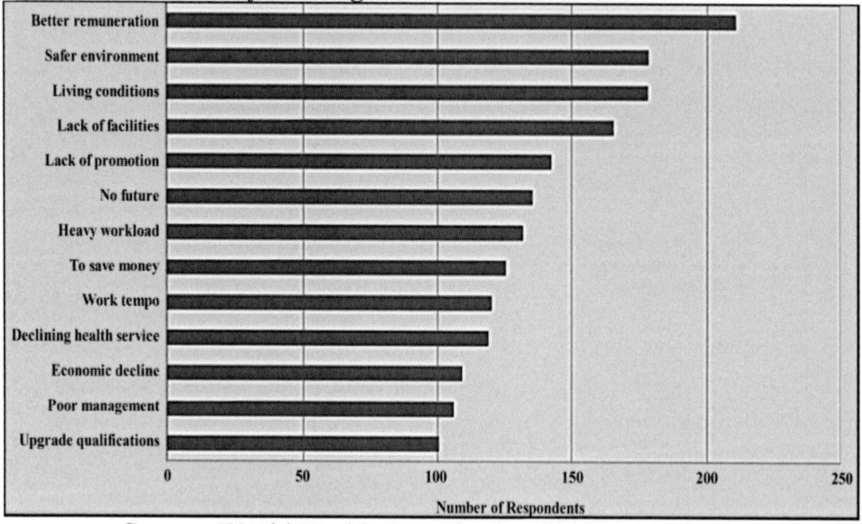


Source: World Health Organisation (WHO) 2006: 99

Firstly, decision-making for migration may result largely from a household, not an individual intention or strategy and gender can make a considerable difference in such collective decision-making processes (UN-DESA 2005). Regarding the migration of overseas nurses, including Malawians, it has been highlighted that in particular older nurses work for *back home*[6] and seek migration as part of a family economic strategy (Larsen et al. 2005; Aboderin 2007).

Secondly, migrant communities and networks may play an essential role in assessing the viability of migration, choosing a destination and organizing a migration project, as has been

[6] The expressions *back home* and *home country* differ from the more often used technical terms *source country* and *country of origin* in suggesting a strong social relatedness between the migrant and his or her national community as a *home*. This suggestion is not necessarily capturing the relation between all migrant nurses and their origin appropriately. Despite acknowledging this weakness, the term *home* will be applied in this study as it was found to reflect the study participants' referencing and reasoning about Malawi more adequately than the common technical terms.

documented e.g. for Indian and Filipina nurses in the UK (Alonso-Garbayo and Maben 2009). Establishing transnational social spaces, they shape the social perception and imagination of migration as a cultural attribute, strengthening the continuity of migration flows over time and instituting migration as a community value. Migration comes to be perceived as a common biographic *rite of passage*, which the coming generations are expected to go through as well.

"At the community level, migration becomes deeply ingrained into the repertoire of people's behaviors, and values associated with migration become part of the community's values. For young men, and in many settings young women as well, migration becomes a *rite of passage*, and those who do not attempt to elevate their status through international movement are considered lazy, unenterprising, and undesirable." (Massey et al. 1993: 493, emphasis C.V.)

Thirdly, South-North migration is oftentimes shaped by the historical experiences and relationships of colonialism and by images about the *developed* as compared to the *developing* world. Imperial history and colonial ties have been elicited as important backgrounds e.g. in understanding the culture and conditions of nurse's migration from the Philippines (Schultheiss 2010; Alonso-Garbayo and Maben 2009). Grigulis has illustrated the links between nurse migration and the social and political situation during different historical periods in postcolonial Malawi, pointing to the limitation of any migration model to the conditions of a specific socio-political context given at a particular point in time (Grigulis 2010).

Lastly, from individual stories of motivations, expectations and reasons for migration, an abundance of intangible constellations emerges, interweaving structural factors with the individual biography (age/life stage, social and cultural provenience, lifestyle, self-identities and future visions) into an imagination about the benefits of migration. In an attempt to categorize these individual constellations, Kingma (2006) has distinguished five types of migrant nurses: economic migrants (attracted by better standard of living), quality of life migrants (interested in safety and well-being), career move migrants (motivated by enhanced career opportunities), partner migrants (following their partner) and adventure migrants (using their nursing qualifications to finance travel to a destination country to gain new experiences).

Regarding the patterns of international migration, research has highlighted that the enormous variety and complexity of migration flows questions the usefulness of general migration theories in predicting them. Among the dynamics complicating classical models of migration are global migration chains, temporary and permanent return migration, remigration and transnationalism (Arango 2000; UNFPA 2006; Haour-Knipe and Davies 2008). The concept of *transnationalism* refers to the social dynamics and flows of information and resources that establish between migrants and their communities of origin. It aims to account for the various directionalities of migrant identities and social spheres of reference, as well as for causes and consequences of migration that may not be localized in one country or in another but emerge from spaces of inbetweenness (Luethi 2005). Figure 2 (next page) shows interlinkages of migration flows of health workers for the case of South Africa. It highlights the chain character and multidirectionality of migration and points out that the UK - the main recipient country of South African as well as Malawian nurses – may as well be a country of transition or temporary migration as a permanent destination (Kingma 2006; Buchan et al. 2006).

In the context of the migration of women occupied as care workers (nursing, caring for the elderly, nannying etc.), the concept of *care chains* describes that gaps left behind by women migrants are often refilled by female care workers from other, usually less wealthy countries. In this dynamic, the negative effects of female migration accumulate in poorer countries while hierarchies of gender and class are reproduced and globalized (UNFPA 2006; Smith and Mackintosh 2007). Though some dimensions of this concept apply more closely to the context of unqualified care work, the existence of care chains between nurses e.g. from Malawi, South Africa and the U.K. is a documented phenomenon, through which the social effects of global nurse migration are passed on to poorer countries (JLI 2004).

*Figure 2. Main Channels of Health Workers' International Migration to/out of South Africa*

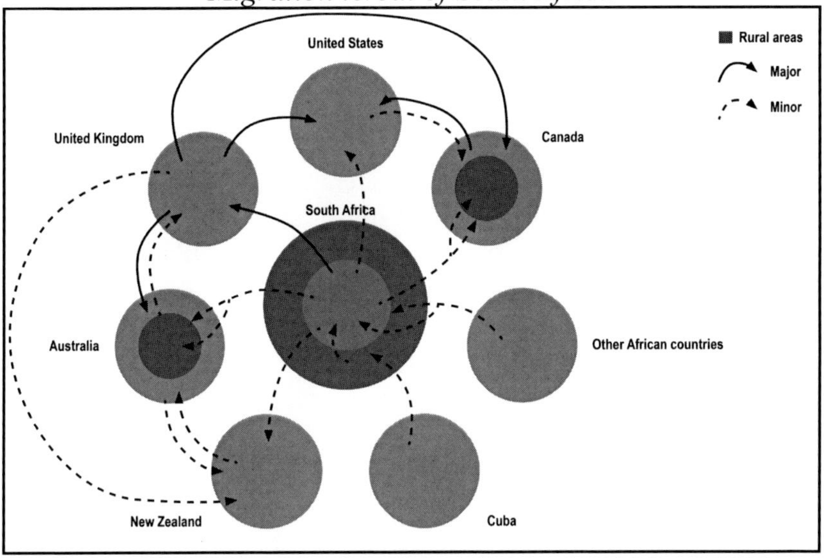


Source: JLI 2004: 104, adapted from Dumont and Meyer 2004

Dynamics of remigration, chain migration, temporary return and transnational activity that may e.g. be related to historical or biographical factors, transnationalism or living conditions and political factors, are often not considered in structural models of health workers' migration such as the national health system perspective described above. However, these dynamics may likewise shape actual migration flows of health workers decisively.

## The Malawian Context

### *Malawi's Health Workforce Shortage*

Malawi's health workforce is far too small for the country's fast-growing population. The last official health workforce census counted 2,932 qualified nurses/midwives and 190 physicians for a population of approximately 13 million (CSR 2007).

The WHO estimates that at least 2.5 physicians, nurses and midwives per 1,000 people are needed to provide adequate primary health care, ignoring the increasing demand in countries with high burden of disease (WHO 2006). With on average 3,050 people per nurse (CSR 2007), that is a nurse to population ratio of ~0,33:1,000, Malawi is among the countries with a most severe health worker shortage, both in global and regional comparison. There are huge inner-country variations with rural districts in Northern Malawi facing the worst coverage situation, counting as little as 0,15 nurses per 1,000 people in Kasungu (CSR 2007) and 51% of the population of Chipita living farer than 8km from the next health centre (MoH 2011b).

The shortage of health personal therefore constitutes a major constraint to the improvement of health care and the achievement of health related development goals. A coverage of the health needs - e.g. for HIV/AIDS related treatment, maternal and child health, and an Essential Health Package meant to grant the poor access to basic care - would require a mayor increase in the health workforce, in particular of nurses (McCoy, McPake and Mwapasa 2008; Joint Learning Initiative 2004).

International migration represents only one among several factors of Malawi's health workforce crisis, next to low and unstable training rates, high attrition and an insufficient number of established posts. The high number of unfilled positions for medical and nursing specialists results mainly from low training capacities, while the high vacancy rate on ministerial level (77% in 2003) is attributed to non-transparent and complicated recruitment procedures in the first place (RoM et al. 2007).

While death continues to be the main factor of attrition since 1994, resignation has increased substantially since 1996 (Figure 3). This development falls together with the liberalization of the health sector that opened new occupational choices to health workers (GoM and UNDP 2002). Today internal migration to private health providers, international organisations and other economic branches beyond health is acknowledged to be a major factor of attrition from the public health service and raises more attention than international migration (Mkwinda-Nyasulu and Chilemba 2007; Grigulis 2010): in 2007 66% out of the 253 health workers employed in NGOs and 60% of the health workers in private health organisations had been recruited from the government sector (CSR 2007).

*Figure 3. Causes of Attrition among MoH Personnel*

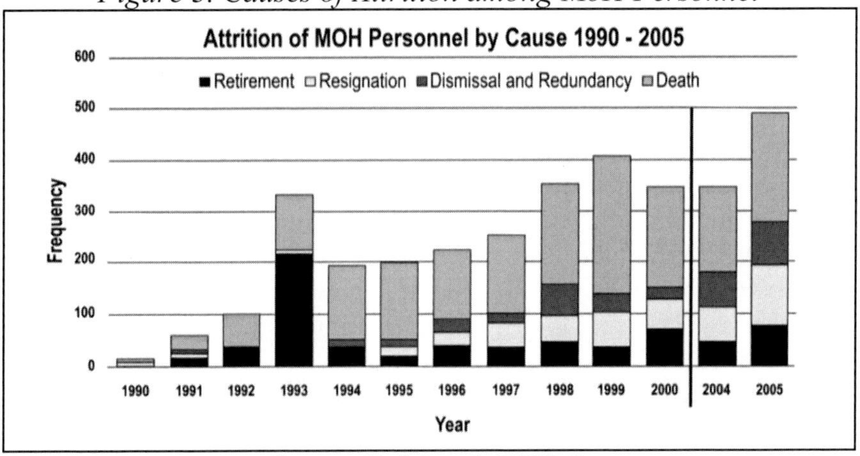


Source: RoM et al. 2007: 3

International NGOs, UN institutions and technical assistance agencies are ambiguous players in this field: on the one hand their agendas are often addressing the public human resources for health shortage, on the other hand they have been accused of poaching actively among highly qualified health workers from public agencies, for whom the salary difference constitutes a major pull-factor. Health workers who resign from public services tend to do so very early in their professional life - after an average of 4.4 years of duty

(CSR 2007). The Malawian Health SWAp-Initiative therefore suggested implementing a Memorandum of Understanding, limiting salary differences and prohibiting poaching to address these detrimental effects (RoM et al. 2007).

In response to the human resource for health crisis, an Emergency Human Resources Programme (EHRP) was put in place from 2004 to 2010 as a joint initiative of the Ministry of Health and partnering development agencies, in particular DFID, the Global Fund, NORAD, GDC as well as the World Bank, UNFPA and UNICEF. Within its five areas of action the programme tackled recruitment (domestic training capacities, international volunteers), retention (monetary and other incentives, professional development) and management aspects of the shortage (human resources monitoring and planning capacity) (Palmer 2006). According to DFID the interventions proved successful to raise the number of nurses in service by 39% (DFID 2010).

However, designed as an emergency programme, some of its approaches were successful to bring fast improvements on the recruitment and retention side, but the introduced measures were cost-intensive and difficult to sustain, despite the relatively high health expenditure of the Malawian government. Experienced difficulties to maintain salary top-ups and training scholarships for health workers in 2009 and 2010 indicated that the conservation of progresses depends largely on continued external funding. [7]

Lamentably, in autumn 2013 the so-called *cashgate* financial corruption scandal threatened the international health funding dramatically. Though the Ministry of Health was not directly implicated, the extensive misappropriation of funds intrusted to the government led to partly temporary, partly ultimate suspensions of international health funding that had been allocated to the government's health budget (e.g. DFID 2015). In view of the economic and political crisis faced between 2010 and 2014, Malawi's ongoing economic vulnerability due to its dependency on agricultural

[7] Between 2008 and 2014 19,4% of the General Government Expenditure went into Government Expenditure on Health. The contribution of NGOs in the same time span equaled 9,6% of the General Government Expenditure (WHO 2014).

production threatened by climate change and volatile export markets, it is not foreseeable that Malawi's health system could overcome its dependency on fluctuating international aid.

### *Nursing in Malawi*

Given that nurses are the mainstay of health care provision in the country, they have been trained in higher number than other cadres and serve at the bedside as well as in the management of health facilities. Where physicians are unavailable, nurses carry far more responsibility for the actual provision of health services then in the European context: it is not uncommon that experienced and well-qualified nursing staff[8] are overseeing the management of whole hospitals, especially in rural areas.

Between 2004 and 2010, large investment by the government and diverse donors to train and retain more nurses achieved a positive trend in the countrywide nurse to population ratio from 0,25:1,000 (2004) to 0,40:1,000 (2009) (DFID 2010). However, since then the vacancy rates continued to be alarming (MoH 2011b). In 2012 74% of the established posts for nursing were still vacant and nurse midwife technicians remained the cadre with the largest staffing gap also in 2014 (MoH 2015).

Research findings on the employment preferences of registered nurses suggest that nurses weigh a considerable variety of factors when making employment choices, including (frequently) net monthly pay, the availability of material resources, and workload, (often) opportunities to upgrade qualifications, place of work, provision of housing, access to in-service training, promotion prospects, grade structure, and transport, and (seldom) health risks (incl. HIV/AIDS), the competency of the administration, supervision, challenges of managing junior members of staff, job security/leave entitlements, and pensions. The chronic shortage of staff in Malawi's public health care centres, low and often irregularly paid salaries paired with promotion systems lacking transparency,

---

[8] The Malawian nursing workforce is divided into registered nurses (cadres trained at degree level or well experienced nurses) and enrolled nurses (lower cadres trained at diploma level). (See Annex Table 2)

and a generally overburdened health care system in terms of a lack of adequate facilities, medical equipment and medications available to treat patients successfully, have accumulated creating a working environment that is highly dissatisfactory to many nurses. (Mangham 2007; Chimwaza et al. 2014)

Despite the large number and important role of nurses in the local health system, Malawian researchers have pointed to the structurally disadvantaged position of nurses in the hierarchy of medical professions as an "*appendage of medicine*" (ibid. 75), which they attribute to its role as feminized profession confronting a male-dominated clinical workforce and society (ibid.). In Malawi nursing tends to be regarded as a women's profession. Introduced by female missionaries, it is still associated with a religious vocation to care and feminine gender attributes. Till 1984 only women nurses were trained at KCN and today's nursing workforce is still dominated by women, though the proportion of male nurses has risen in younger cohorts.[9] Among physicians the ratio is reverse, reproducing a patriarchal social hierarchy in the hospital setting (Muula, Nyasulu and Msiska 2004a+b).

Yet, when placing nursing within the hierarchy of female professions, a different picture emerges. As a Malawian nursing leader highlighted to me, nursing used to be the only professional option for women seeking higher education and, in turn nurses represented an outstandingly respected class among Malawian women, in particular as educational attendance and achievement are generally highly recognized in the society.[10] The latter is indicated by an overwhelming public demand for further education throughout all strata of the society and relates to considerable advantages from being well educated, as degree holders encounter better chances on the Malawian labour market, reach higher incomes, higher job security and low unemployment (Kadzamira 2003; World Bank 2010).

---

[9] Male nurses represented 11.4% of the nursing workforce in 2007 and are particularly underrepresented in older generations (CSR 2007).

[10] Personal communication with Dorothy Ngoma (NONM) in 2010; similarly stated by Grigulis (2010).

Due to the overall conditions of the countries' schooling system, the social exclusivity of education and the competition of Malawians for access and attainment in education continue to be high. Despite the successful introduction of free compulsory primary education in 1994, the enrolment in secondary education, especially among girls, continues to be highly selective by their families' socioeconomic condition (World Bank 2004). Additionally, girls are still heavily under-represented at the level of secondary education and beyond (Figure 4). Despite the dominant share of women in nursing, the University of Malawi estimated the overall female enrolment at 35% in 2009 (UNIMA 2010).[11] Particularly women's participation in science professions is low (Gomile-Chidyaonga 2003; Maluwa-Banda 2004; Ngwira, Kamchedzera and Semu 2003) and gender images about male intellectual superiority continue to shape female self-identities, constraining the chances of girls' educational attainment in Malawi (Davison 1993; Kamwendo 2010, Chimomombo et al. 2000).

In view of the low rate of upper secondary completion and taking into account the high quality differences between different types of secondary schools, the group of nurses approached in this study counts with privileged conditions: almost all participating students[12] stated to have received secondary education in government day, -boarding, mission or private schools, i.e. institutions with higher teaching quality and often higher costs involved.[13]

---

[11] The political representation of women is even weaker and decreasing (Kayuni 2017): despite being headed by a female president for two years, the share of women members in the Malawian Parliament dropped from 22% in 2009 to 16,7% in 2014 (Kayuni 2017, IPU 2015).

[12] Except 6 missing answers

[13] The reputation of government boarding and mission schools as well as selected private schools is particularly high and usually involves a formal selection process. Admission to mission and private schools usually requires the payment of considerable school fees (World Bank 2004).

*Figure 4. Access to and Completion of the Different School Levels by Gender*

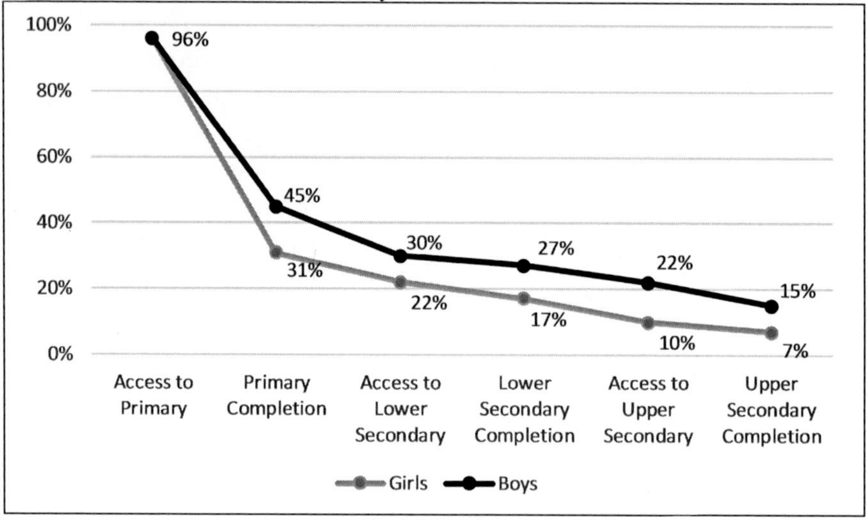


Source: World Bank 2010: 104

Overall, the economic status of the family reflects closely in the educational attainment of children in the Malawi School Certificate of Education (MSCE) examinations, the precondition to enter tertiary education (Lewin and Sayed 2005; World Bank 2004; Kadzamira 2003). The admission to tertiary education, in particular to the public university UNIMA, is highly competitive among MSCE performers as is commonly recognized among Malawians.

In this light, higher education such as the nursing degree programme becomes a distinctive resource that remains exclusive to a small, socioeconomically advantaged group of people who make use of it to increase their capacity of raising and reproducing socioeconomic profits and an elevated social status. Within the hierarchy of Nursing in Malawi, degree nurses represent a cadre of elevated, yet in their working environment often contested status. Young degree nurses in Malawi are thus necessarily drawn into a vague and ambivalent position between educational privilege, symbolical status and precariousness in the professional day-to-day practice.

### *Malawian (Nurses') History of Migration*

As both the history of Malawi and the history of nursing in the country have been shaped by labour migration throughout many years, historical experiences build a subtle ground for the formation of a social imagination of migration that is to be considered as an important backdrop for young nurses' premature images and intentions of migrating in future.

Professional nursing care came to Malawi as to other colonies with the immigration of white female missionaries as part of the British colonial invasion, transporting on behalf of nursing the racist images and values of a *Western* superiority and establishing nursing as a prestigious profession linked to *Western civilization*[14]. In South Africa the colonial administrations later allowed local women to train as nurses, driven by the idea to enforce racial segregation in nursing and to institute a new class of black, *civilized* womanhood (Schultheiss 2011). In Malawi, the colonial administration did not engage in a local training of nurses but picked a small selection of women to train in nursing colleges in Britain. This early migration was perceived as a privilege and brought those selected a high professional status and respect for their experience back in Malawi (Grigulis 2010). While the foundation of the University of Malawi dates back to the year of independence (1964), a nursing degree remained bound to a move abroad until 1979 (foundation of KCN), a career as physician until 1991 (foundation of the College of Medicine COM) (UNIMA 2010). The most important authority of the country throughout more that 20 years, Malawi's first president Dr. Hastings Kamuzu Banda, had been one of those who had enjoyed the privilege to train and work as a physician in the UK. Today's nursing college is

---

[14] This emphasis means to remind that the historical invention of the concepts *the West* and *Western civilization* as well as the usage of these concepts are highly problematic: inherent to them are essentialist and racialized ideas of European cultural superiority and development and legitimizations of imperialism. For a critical genesis of the concept see for example Bonnett (2003). When using the term in the following, I imply this problematic connotation.

named after him and he remains highly respected among many Malawian nurses till present days (Grigulis 2010).

This background of nursing in Malawi points to the intertwining of the high local status of the nursing profession with migration and the idea of acquiring access to *Western civilization*. It suggests the early development of a tradition of nurse migration, connected with the establishment of a migrant community and the evolution of a "culture of migration" (Massey et al. 1998: 47-48) for purposes of professional training.

> "As migration grows in prevalence within a community, it changes values and cultural perceptions in ways that increase the probability of future migration. […] At the community level, migration becomes deeply ingrained into the repertoire of people's behaviors, and values associated with migration become part of the community's values." (Massey et al. 1998: 47)

A vivid *culture of migration* in the community of Malawian nurses would imply that socially transmitted migration aspirations inscribe into the individuals' migration projects and practices of concern in this study, and shape in return the common repertoire of perceptions and aspirations in the young generation of nursing.

While the culture of nurse migration and the imperial mission of nursing care have a female face, the wider *culture of migration* in Malawi is male-dominated. A brief review of migration from Malawi reveals a massive scale and importance of male labour migration to South Africa, established as a form of colonial exploitation by the British colonial rule and persisting until the late 1980s. Labour migration established within Southern Africa as a symptom of colonial-capitalist modes of production raising the need for labour supply in centres of colonial exploitation economy - on farms, in mines and in manufacturing industries. The colonial administration did not suspect Malawi to hold marketable natural resources and thus, instead of exploiting commodities, depopulated rural areas to exploit Malawian men's labour force in Rhodesia and South Africa (Weyl 1980). Though this is considered to have had strong negative implications on economic development and subsistence agriculture in Malawi (Weyl 1980), Labour migration became popular as wage labour in South African mines generated higher income than the work on Malawian farms, which received most of their labour supply from Mozambique. This way, large-scale male migration established over the years in the Malawian society as a common livelihood strategy, connected with a social repertoire of perceptions integrating economic chances and personal dangers of migration. While the economic importance of migration from Malawi is confirmed, its historical-sociological consequences remain largely unexplored.

A Malawian census in 2008, capturing recent trends in non-return migration between 1998 and 2008, reveals continuity in that non-return migration remains to be dominated by young males (average sex ratio 5:1) with South Africa as most important destination country (NSO 2010). As the census categories of studying, mine and farm work or official business captured less than 40% of the non-return migrants, the classical areas of occupation abroad however seem to have lost importance towards different other low-status jobs, as the authors suspect.

The census points to the increasing importance of long-term migration for study purposes, implying a growing inclination towards early migration and migration of the highly skilled. Muula (2006) estimates that most migrating health professionals leave Malawi within the first 5 years after graduation. In contrast, Palmer (2006) and Buchan et al. (2006) observed the high participation of older, well-experienced nurses in international migration from Malawi and Southern African Countries in general.

Given the low participation of women in non-return migration from Malawi in general, their share in medical migration is outstanding with 40% between 2004-08. Furthermore, women migrants are more strongly represented among students (25%) than among overall migrants (16%) (NSO 2010 for the years 2004-08), and more inclined to leave at a young age as well as to go overseas.[15] This clearly suggests an importance of global nurse migra-

[15] According to the census, more than 40% of all not yet returned overseas migrants were female and the share of overseas-migrants in overall female non-return migrants amounted to 19%, as compared to 6% for males.

tion from Malawi, be it as a form of labour or student migration or beyond, under a gender and migration perspective.

### *Migration Trends among Malawian Nurses since 2000*

Taking a health system perspective, it is of foremost importance to acknowledge the relativity of small numbers: in Malawi's understaffed health service already a very modest migration of nurses has a strong weight. Clemens and Patterson (2008) found 377 Malawian born nurses in the censuses of the main recipient countries by the year 2000, amounting to 17% of Malawi's overall domestic health workforce of 1999. Far most of these nurses had settled in the USA and the UK (171 each). In 2002, when 75 Malawian nurses newly registered with the UK Nurses and Midwives Council (UK NMC) this accounted for a further loss of almost 12% of Malawi's overall domestic nursing workforce (Ross, Polsky and Solchasky 2005). By comparison, the UK NMC counted in the same year 183 registrations of nurses from the neighbour state Zambia with a population similar to the Malawian, however this represented only 2% of Zambia's overall nursing workforce (ibid.).

Reviewing the recent outmigration trend among Malawian nurses between 2000 and 2010, the registers of the Nurses and Midwives Council of Malawi (NMCM) and the UK (UK NMC) suggest that the peek years of migration were from 2000 and 2005, when a sharp, persistent decline manifests. Throughout this period the UK have been the envisaged destination of far most Malawian nurses when seeking registration to go abroad: 148 of 240 registrants at the NMCM from 01/2004 to 11/2010 named the UK as envisaged destination (NMCM 2010a). The ebbing of registrations in 2006 goes largely to the account of the diminution of applicants for the UK, which is confirmed by the UK NMC data (UK NMC 2008 and 2011). The NMCM recorded fluctuant small-scale registrations for the ZAR (5-8 annual registrations between 2007 and 2009) and the USA, other South African countries (esp. Botswana) as well as North American and European countries (between 2007 and 2010 up to 3 annual registrations). The registration data suggests that lower nursing cadres as well as male nurses are relatively underrepresented in official nurse migration.[16]

These often-cited figures of the NMCM need to be put into perspective taking into account its constraints as a data source far from appropriate to give a reliable picture of the scale and destinations of outmigration. It is only due to the lack of comprehensive data that research is obliged to relate to the so-called register for "Certificates of Good Standing" held by the NMCM. The manually kept books of the Council's registration office document each nurse who ordered and received such a certificate, which is required to register with an NMC in the prospective destination country and obtain the permit necessary to practice as a qualified nurse there (NMCM 2010b).

The low quality of this source became obvious to me in a review of the books for the period 2004-2010, finding that it was prone to double-counting and incomplete information. The brilliant memory of the office employee (in-charge of the registrations since many years) amended the books with important insights. The register does not inform about the current country of residence of the applicant, including nurses who had left years ago already for family reunification and the like. The registrar furthermore advised me that throughout the peak years it was popular among nursing graduates to register prematurely, in order to be prepared if chances would show (NMCM 2010b). Thus, next to different technical constraints, the serious limitation of this register is that it serves merely to give an idea of the *migration potential* among nurses, while it does not indicate outmigration rates. The data has been misinterpreted severally in this regard, e.g. by DFID (2010), treating the numbers as real migration rate and Mangham (2007: 6) citing the same numbers as "number of registered nurses that have left Malawi and subsequently sought validation of their qualifications".

[16] Between 2004 and 2010 less than 3% of the applicants for a Certificate of Good Standing were male, less than 1/4 enrolled nurses (NMCM 2010a). In 2007 male nurses represented 11,4%, enrolled nurses 1/3 of the nursing workforce (RoM et al. 2007).

A comparison of the numbers held by the NMCs of Malawi and the UK may therefore roughly inform on the difference between sought and realized migration throughout the peak years of nurse migration to the UK. As Figure 5 shows, the NMCM data overestimates outmigration of nurses by far. The progressions are hardly comparable, in particular when considering the time difference of minimum one year between the registrations.[17] The overall scope of registrations differs by more than 25% throughout the period. Though registrations by the UK NMC can be regarded as the more viable estimate of actual nurse migration, they may also be misleading in some cases: as the findings of Grigulis (2010) suggest, nurses went as far as registering in the UK but then failed to migrate or, on the contrary, left Malawi but failed to register, taking up other care occupations instead.

*Figure 5. Registrations of Malawian Nurses to Work in the UK*

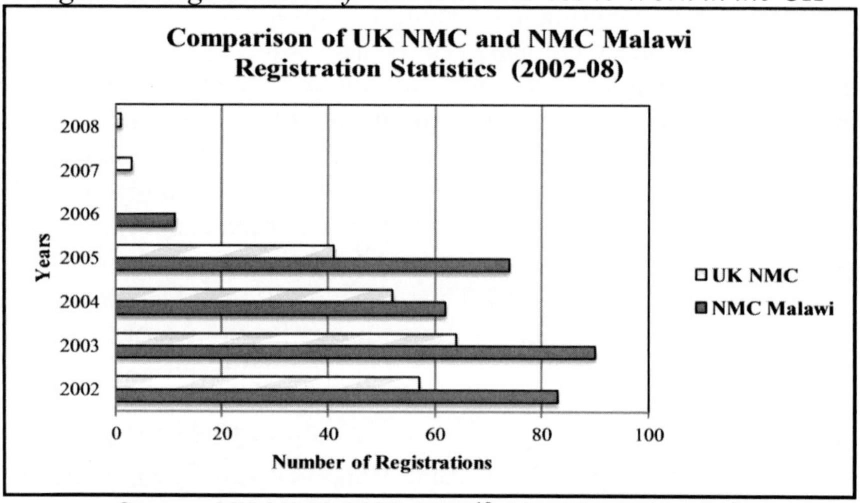


Source: UK NMC 2003-2008[18]; NMCM 2010a+b[19]

[17] A time difference of one year between the registrations is to be considered until 2006. After that year, registration defers by approximately two years, as overseas nurses are since obliged to comply an Overseas Nursing Programme before being admitted to register.

[18] Initial admissions to the UK overseas register between march 2002 and march 2009 (statistical year from march till march).

In an aura of urgency, the sharp decrease of Malawian nurses' registrations to work in the UK has been overlooked at first by some research (e.g. Mangham 2007). When trying to make sense of the apparent decline, the literature gives different reasons. Optimistic voices attribute some of it to Malawi's improved HRH policies, in particular the monetary incentive of salary top-ups (DFID 2010; Tambulasi and Chasukwa 2011). A further factor might have been the implementation of ethical frameworks for the recruitment of health workers from developing countries: the UK NHS adapted its recruitment policies in recent years to control and restrict the private recruitment of nurses, following the ethical recruitment guidelines of a Code of Practice and focusing instead on bilateral agreements with India, the Philippines and South Africa (Buchan and McPake 2007). While the Code of Practice has been set as a binding measure for the UK National Health Services (NHS) and, since 2004, for all private sector organisations providing services to the NHS (DoH UK 2004), it is not able to regulate recruitment in the private health sector. South Africa, another important destination for nurses from Malawi throughout the peak years of international migration, is taking a similar approach as the UK (ZAR 2002+2010). However, countries like the USA still rely on active recruitment via private agencies, even in countries like Malawi (Ngoma in VSO 2010).

Another explanation for the decrease concerns developments on the UK's nursing labour market, where the demand for overseas nurses fell in 2006 due to high numbers of domestic graduates and financial cutbacks of public health services. For nurses from countries without bilateral agreements these circumstances affect the conditions for labour migration to the UK sensitively, as they are since facing new barriers such as a restrictive issuing of work permits, additional language and skill test requirements and an

[19] First registrations identified during a personal manual review and revision of the register. Differences between this data and NMCM data cited in other studies go back to double counts, renewals or repetitive applications in the original register.

"UK/European Economic Area nationals first" employment policy (Buchan and McPake 2007).

Interestingly, the decline of Malawian nurses' migration suggested by the professional registers reviewed above does not reflect in the Malawian census data 2008 for migrants in the health field. Since 2006, the applications of women nurses at the NMCM are exceeded increasingly by the census numbers for female non-return migrants occupied in health with 35:19 in 2006, 62:13 in 2007, and 38 (half year):16 (whole year) in 2008 (NSO 2009). While the two data sources are of course not directly compatible, the census' findings call into question whether outmigration of women to work in the health sector, eventually including registered nurses and other qualified health workers, has decreased as much as expected. They raise the concern that female health workers might be leaving without registering, that *care drain* might now drift through more informal and precarious channels, and that countries, job positions and occupational sectors such as private home care with less restrictive registration procedures might be gaining importance. This would, in turn, affect migrating nurses' prospects to meet the historically grown expectations in the Malawian society to generate privilege and status in the course of migration.

Further questions on the professional registration statistics emerge from destination countries' censuses (Clemens and Patterson 2008): the equal representation of Malawian nurses in the 2000 censuses of the UK and the USA would have raised the expectation to find a stronger share of applicants destining the USA, especially as US recruitment agencies are suspected to continue practicing in Malawi. Informal labour migration of Malawian nurses as well as remigration from e.g. the UK might be of relevance in this context, too.

### *Patterns of Nurse Migration from Malawi*

Beyond the flows, the patterns of nurses' migration from Malawi are of relevance to this study and its interest in biographical aspects of nurse migration. Despite the noteworthy symbolic history of Malawian nurses migration, the perspective driving most research on the topic has so far been narrowly policy-oriented, identifying in particular health system related push and pull factors of migration (Mkwinda-Nyasulu and Chilemba 2007), or quantifying the phenomenon and its economic impact and discussing applicable political solutions (Muula 2006a-c; Muula, Panulo and Maseko 2006; Muula and Maseko 2006; Manafa et al. 2009). More recently, Tambulasi and Chasukwa (2011) have added an evaluation of existing measures to hold the medical *brain drain*.

Professional push factors for the *brain drain* of nurses and other health professionals in Malawi have been found in high workload, low salaries, and poor working conditions regarding equipment and safety, leading to moral distress, frustration or burnout (Tambulasi and Chasukwa 2011). Several studies have furthermore pointed to Malawian health workers, in particular nurses' thirst for professional development and further education as a factor for migration (Muula and Maseko 2006; Mangham 2007; Mkwinda-Nyasulu and Chilemba 2007). Main push factors included:

„[…] higher wages and income, higher standard of living, better working conditions; job and career opportunities and professional development, substantial funds for research, advanced technology, modern facilities, availability of experienced support staff, political stability, modern educational system, prestige of 'foreign training', meritocracy, transparency, and intellectual freedom.“ (Tambulasi and Chasukwa 2011: 19)

According to this most recent study, internal and external *brain drain* are increasingly becoming a concern among highly qualified health professionals due to push factors within the administration of the health system, in particular ambiguous prospects to advance one's job position due to unclear career paths, little opportunity to apply specialist capacities, and delayed or absent promotion in salary and position:

“ '[…] the more specialized people are, the high [sic.] are chances that they will leave government. Reasons being that they fell [sic.] they are not being recognized by their new qualifications and promotions take longer. You are lucky if you get promoted in three years after the specialization training.' " (Interviewed MoH official in ibid.: 19)

With regard to degree nurses the difficulty to come into leading functions despite holding higher qualifications is highlighted as a particular concern:

„[…] nurses do not normally head institutions despite them having a degree. In most cases health centers are headed by diploma level clinical officers or certificate level medical assistants and this frustrates the degree nurse. As one of them hinted 'even if you hold masters degree and you go to a health center you cannot head it.' " (Ibid. 19).

While these studies indirectly hint at wider biographic concerns of professional and social status as possible roots of decisions to migrate, the researchers' focus on structural problems of the Malawian public health system leads them to a rather simplistic general analysis of the issue, suggesting that the health system's low capacity to compete against occupational environments elsewhere was the main if not only relevant background of medical migration.

The existing research on nurse migration suffers furthermore from a bias towards the emigration side. This inclination is plausible in view of the political concern about the effects of health workers' *brain drain* and the assumption that the Malawian nursing sector is situated at the end of a labour migration chain, meaning that outmigration is not replaced but leaving a care gap. Indeed, there is no evidence that the in majority female lifetime-immigrants to Malawi (NSO 2010) would engage in the nursing field.

However, a comparison of numbers cited by DFID (2010) and the NMCM registers (2010a) reveals that international nursing volunteers coming to Malawi outnumbered Malawian nurses seeking to work abroad between 2006 and 2010. In 2003 the Medical Council of Malawi (MCM) registered 252 doctors of whom 51.2% were Malawian and 48.8% non-Malawian. Only 35.7% of the doctors had obtained their initial medical education in Malawi (Muula 2006a). In 2009 265 physicians were practising in Malawi, however more than a forth of them were international volunteers (DFID 2010). While the contribution of international volunteers and medical education abroad is documented, it remains neglected in studies on the migration of health workers in Malawi. Even less visible is the return migration of nurses, which has not been recorded at all, making it impossible to build nurses returning into the Malawian health service into the picture.[20] The narrow focus of migration records and studies on supposedly non-return emigration has left a considerable knowledge gap on the role of international volunteers and the potential health gains connected to an unknown number of migrant nurses returning into service, eventually even with crucial additional qualifications obtained abroad.

Beyond the immediate political concerns with Malawi's health workforce crisis, Malawian nurses' personal approaches to migration have gained little attention. The only exception to this is the dissertation of Grigulis (2010), which gives a detailed insight into the individual and socio-historical dimensions of migration intentions and biographic decisions of previous generations of Malawian nurses. Her exploration of reasons and patterns of migration in different generations of Malawian nurses and changing presidential periods reveals remarkable shifts in the motivations to migrate, relating to the overall socio-political situation in Malawi, the local employment and working conditions for nurses and the global conditions to migrate.

Her findings suggest that nurses in the presidential period of President Bingu wa Mutharika from 2004 till 2012 faced difficulties to enter the UK labour market and therefore expected international migration to be less feasible. Instead, they tended towards inner-country occupational alternatives, in particular posts in NGOs (Grigulis 2010). Grigulis identifies a changing backdrop of young nurses' intentions to migrate, rooted in a generational shift of nurses' professional motivation from admiration, pride in having a nurse in the family and wanting to care for Malawians among nurses graduated before 2000, towards obtaining qualifications and

---

[20] Professional registers in Malawi do not include this information and the register of nurses working in Malawi is not connected to the register of nurses who applies to work abroad, making it impossible to identify returnees systematically.

finding marketable career prospects (Grigulis, Prost and Osrin 2009). Her evaluation of push and pull factors of Malawian nurse migration adds the role of conditions external to the health system to the picture, pointing to different enabling factors of migration, survival strategies of the family, social appreciation for migration, the impact of a migration trend among nurses, as well as lifestyle-related expectations towards the destination country (Figure 6).

### *Conclusions*

An analysis of the role of migration in individual biographies and life scripts of Malawian nurses requires being able to link to broad range of possibly relevant meanings and contexts of nurse migration. In this chapter, I have therefore attempted to introduce nurse migration from Malawi as a complex phenomenon in which a historic legacy of migration and nursing as a status profession comes to interweave with todays globalizing market for health workers, high expectations towards the benefits of education and a Malawian health system in precarious state, causing highly unsatisfactory working conditions. These different angles of the situation of nurses in Malawi reveal the ambiguity of young nurses' position between privilege and disadvantage, creating a shaky ground for their future outlook and likely raising biographical dilemmas related to migration, which are addressed and negotiated as part of the individual life scripts and life plans.

*Figure 6. Push- and Pull-factor Model of Malawian Nurse Migration*

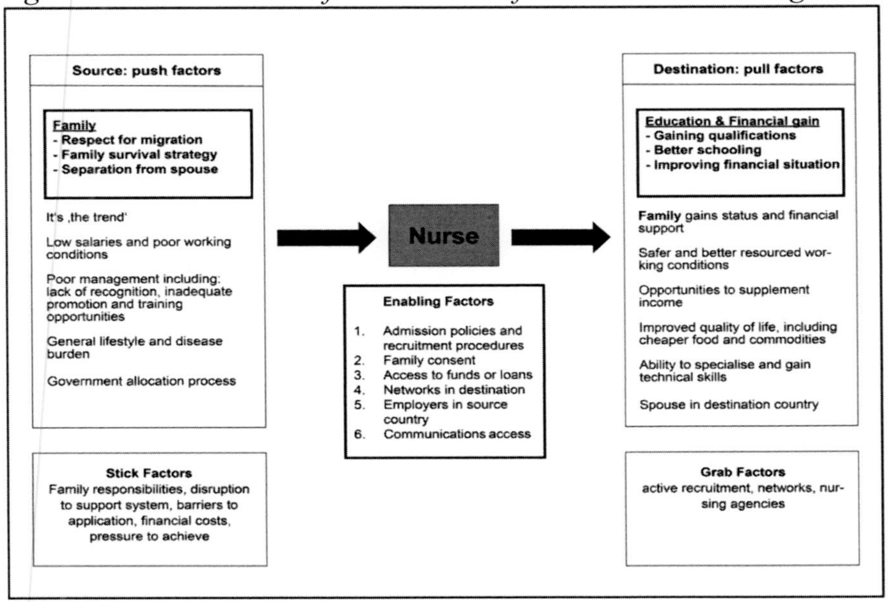


Source: Grigulis 2010: 263

# III. THE RESEARCH PROJECT

## The Study Design

The study at the centre of this book targets the migration projects young nursing graduates from Malawi are developing as part of their future visions and personal life scripts. It aims to contribute to the body of literature on nurse migration in the context of Malawi and beyond, exploring for the case of young nurses the qualities of migration intentions as a step in life-decision-making, and disentangling as well as examining the ways different personal, social and occupational factors of migration decision-making interrelate. Its central objective is to scrutinize and analyse young Malawian Bachelor of Nursing graduates' personal reasoning on and early intentions of migration as part of their life planning and self-perceptions. In this attempt, life scripts, self-identities and migration outlooks are tracked in students' biographical background, career decision-making, gender images and social environment, and analysed against the background of globalization and *(post)colonial*[1] imaginations.

Data collection and analysis were guided by the following research questions: How far are migration intentions relevant to the life planning of students with a degree in nursing? Which collective experiences and ideas of migration, which life scripts and self-identities generate this relevance and how? As the study was conducted within the field of International Development Studies and in cooperation with the Gesellschaft für Internationale Zusammenarbeit (GIZ) the findings were evaluated regarding their impact on development policy, following a third research question: which consequences arise from these findings for the design of

---

[1] The spelling *postcolonial* is used when neutrally referring to the time after colonialism, the spelling *post-colonial* when referring to the school of thought of post-colonial studies and the spelling *(post)colonial* when referring to repercussions of colonial images and conditions beyond the time of colonialism or till today.

development policies to improve the retention of nurses for the Malawian health system and the *brain gain* from nurses' migration?

The sampling of research participants was not directed by the aim to select a representative group of students and would, in view of the exploratory approach, ideally have been a theoretical sample, including in the first place nurses with as many different biographical perspectives on migration as possible and later selecting participants according to theoretically relevant features. A broad sample of nurses from different cadres would have meant to approach nurses situated in very different professional and social environments, associated with different expectations and motivations towards migration. However, accounting for the available resources and the time frame to conduct this study, a more focused population of research was indicated to allow for an in-depth analysis. In order to explore specific profiles of nurse migration, other researchers recommended focusing on one specific group of nurses (Alonso-Garbayo and Maben 2009).

Following this line, the study is limited to one selected cadre and cohort of nurses, Bachelor of Nursing graduates at the point of their graduation. It aims at giving a detailed and specific picture of migration intentions within the context of their particular life scripts and social as well as professional conditions. Starting from a convenience sample based on an invitation to all nurses of the graduating cohort to participate in group-discussions, I proceeded towards theoretical sampling when selecting participants for follow-up in-depth interviews. Self-selection processes as well as the theoretically focused interview sampling over-represent those students who felt attracted by the topic of migration or had declared migration intentions. Despite this bias, as almost one third of the 2010 cohort of Bachelor of Nursing graduates participated, the findings refer to a quantitatively considerable subgroup. Therefore, findings for a strong majority of research participants are indicated in quantitative terms as well.

A focus on Bachelor of Nursing graduates is expedient as the migration of nurses with a university degree raises particular concerns among Malawian nursing leaders: high political commitment and investment have been raised to train them, in hopes of filling the pool of highly qualified nurses so urgently on demand (see Annex Table 2). At the same time, graduated nurses count with an internationally recognized academic certificate that improves their professional opportunities abroad. The migration of this cadre has been associated with high vacancy rates in core positions of the care system and with substantial financial losses (Muula, Panulo and Maseko 2006). Grigulis, Prost and Osrin (2009) furthermore observed that the young generation of nursing graduates approach their profession more as a rewarding career than as a vocation, which is thought to affect their motivations to work in the Malawian system negatively as long as migration promises better career opportunities.

The study applies a primarily micro-sociological research perspective, developing its findings from representations and conceptions of future life inherent to individual actors' life planning and concepts of life and self. Individual strategies of action and future aspirations are approached in their associations with and dissociations from social rules and role expectations. Going beyond the individual level of biographical aspirations, this approach seeks to bear contextual insights into young nurses' social environment and collective future outlooks. Structures of the individual life plan and concepts of life and self are thus always explored in their linkage to common life course representations and social dynamics. The choice of methods, combining group and personal settings acknowledges the reciprocal influence of collective and individual perspectives, concrete plans and latent scripts on the students' biographic future perspectives regarding migration.

For the analysis of the data, the Grounded Theory methodology as described by Strauss and Corbin (1990a) as well as Charmaz (2006) was selected, as it is suitable to pursue theory-generating research on the basis of qualitative data and exploratory research designs. Grounded Theory is based on comparison and differentiation of observations on a specific empirical event or phenomenon. Though the approach has received minor attention in development research, the instruments it delivers are particularly apt to deal self-reflectively with the specific difficulties of research in unacquainted settings and (post)colonial contexts (Schultz 2014).

Following the Grounded Theory approach, I analysed the data starting from an open-coding process in which the data is intensively scrutinized for relevant details, which are then named and translated into initial categories. Advancing in different steps from open to more structured axial and selective coding and memo writing, fragments of analysis are developed and more and more encompassing and complex categories formulated. This analytical process aims for the generation of substantive theory of the phenomenon of concern and eventually extends beyond this phenomenon to generalize the findings towards an abstract grounded theory (Strauss and Corbin 1990b). Instead of introducing theoretical points of reference beforehand, these are developed and selected accompanying the data analysis. This approach fits closely with the research context and purpose of this study to broaden the substantial understanding of the phenomenon of migration intentions in a so far little researched biographical context, and to develop grounded anchors for its theoretical understanding. The created codes and memos are based in quotes, reflections on the transcripts, documentations of workshops and interviews and theoretical memos. Theory and literature review accompanied the data analysis.

Taking an explorative, qualitative approach, the research is designed to contribute fundamental qualitative data and analytical concepts on early decision-making for migration among young academic nurses in the (post)colonial Malawian context. It aims to provide comprehensive elements for a wider substantive theory of nurses' migration intentions in Malawi to be pursued by further, more encompassing studies.

## Central Concepts

### *Life Course, Future Plans and Life Scripts*

This study inquires into students' biographic experiences, self-identities and social environments, their collective ideas about migration in the life course and public expectations towards their social group. These different variables are built into the analysis to allow exploring wider contexts of the role of migration in their future plans and life scripts. The students' *biographical horizons* for central life projects are taken as axes for this exploration.

The interpretation of students' life scripts and plans draws on concepts of Pierre Bourdieu and Anthony Giddens, whose theories approach self-identity and life course planning from contradictory points of view: Bourdieu conceptualizes an individual's action as predefined by his or her habitus. Bourdieu defines habitus as the embodying of family and class related experiences with social and economic conditions. The habitus shapes the perceptions about social realities and determines, often unconsciously, the strategies of action that are and can be pursued (Bourdieu 1986). He reveals how life planning and decision-making are marked by the competition of actors in a social field of power, with the aim to stabilize and improve their relative economic capital (control over financial resources), cultural capital (resources linked to the acquisition of knowledge and skills) and social capital (social networks of support and prestige), sanctioned and valued according to the symbolic capital they inherit (their conformity with and status within social norms, legislation and jurisdiction) (Bourdieu 1986 and 1998, Buchmann 1998; Robb et al. 2007). Capital in the sense of Bourdieu means accumulated labour that, in objectified and embodied forms, creates potential "*capacity to produce profits and to reproduce itself in identical and expanded forms*" (Bourdieu 1986: 46). Each individual action can be regarded as an integrated part of the larger activity of organizing one's life, in which strategies of investing accessible resources of cultural or economic capital are organized towards a strategy of action aiming to maximize material and symbolic profits in order to reproduce or enhance the individual's social position (Buchmann 1989 citing Bourdieu).

While Bourdieu's framework emphasizes the congruence of individual action with demands and determining mechanisms of the social environment, Giddens (1991) takes an individualistic approach to identity and decision-making. In Giddens' understanding, the self and the life plan are fragile and reflexive projects. He points to the individuals' power of choice over self-identities, concepts of life and lifestyles in late modern societies. The concept of *late modernity* has been introduced by Giddens to characterize the social dynamics that develop as a reflexive reaction to the emancipatory project of *Western* modernity and globalisation, contrasting a late modern globality with the local contexts of what he calls *traditional* societies. Such bipolar constructions of *Western*/global modernity versus oriental/local traditionalism reflect a problematic Eurocentric thinking (see Footnote 15, p. 26) and have (if used altogether) to be treated with caution. Applying Giddens' concept to the supposedly traditional Malawian context, I challenge the binary mindset and emphasize the interference of a global climate of late modernity within postcolonial societies like the Malawian, generating in the local context dynamics that are specific to late modern globalisation. This approach allows making sense of the interaction of late modern and long-established elements in the identity formation of a generation of nurses that positions in-between global and local realms, and accounts for the students perceptions about lifestyle differences between the global and the local.

The parallel consideration of the opposing theories of Bourdieu and Giddens was found to be enriching to trace the ambivalent influences of collective and individual power in self-identity formation and strategies of action shaping the place of migration in the students' life planning and life script.

Concrete life plans and general scripts of life are the core frame into which student nurses' motivations to migrate are build in this biographical analysis. They bundle the individual priorities, plans and milestones into a story about the imagined future life.

When studying the orienting frames of German women's life decision-making, Keddi (2003; 2008) found that plans were shifting considerably with changing living conditions and life-stages, whereas personal life projects (e.g. of partnership, career, self-actualisation, tradition or overcoming biographic crises) guided the life decision-making fundamentally and consistently over a longer period of time as a *biographical horizon* and subliminal *script of life*. She identifies *life themes* that shape and structure young women's thoughts, feelings, plans and decisions constantly over longer periods of time, outliving even fundamental changes in the professional, social or personal life. This suggests a necessity to differentiate between life plans that are developed, adjusted, amended or abandoned according to experiences, individual orientations and social contexts, and life themes and underlying scripts of life, which are likely to structure the biographical outlook more endurably.

Scripts of life reflect the interaction of individual psychological needs and ambitions with collective concepts of a "*public life course*" (Buchmann 1998: 26). The latter transmits social and cultural rules, values, discourses and conditions, defining what is collectively regarded as a successful life (ibid.; Günther 2008). Buchmann shows in her analysis of youth in the US-American society, how individual scripts of life can be shaped deeply by a *public life course* of social definitions, role as well as status expectations regarding a person's life: the *public life course* of US-American youth reflected in the researched individual life designs and was appropriated to the personal conditions of life (ibid.). The possibilities to integrate the collective and the individual dimensions of the life course into a personal biographical story are partly determined by social concepts of life, collective orientations and a society's openness towards different lifestyles as social points of reference the individual may rely on (ibid.).

Future life plans and scripts of life may serve to display coherence of a biography and self-identity and situate the individual in relation to its social group, responding to the questions "*Where do I/we come from? Who am I/are we? Where do I/we go?*" (translated from Bosse 1999 quoted in Günther 2008: 54). While aiming to secure biographic continuity, every life plan remains grounded in current circumstances, social conditions and living contexts, making its vulnerability to changes obvious.

"[A] self-identity has to be created and more or less continually reordered against the backdrop of shifting experiences of day-to-day life and the fragmenting tendencies of modern institutions." (Giddens 1991: 186)

Shifting and ambiguous identities and self-perceptions can fundamentally influence this (re)writing of the life plan. The postcolonial social context of Malawi entails the conditions for particularly plural and hybrid self-identities, negotiating and integrating (post)colonial experiences of domination and resistance, globalization and modernization. As Bhabha (1996) notes from a constructivist point of view, post-colonial[27] identity itself is multifaceted, incorporating and reshaping experiences of colonial domination and resistance, and constructing or reconstructing the self in hybrid spaces of in-betweenness and ambiguity. In the absence of a strict value and role system the modern individual itself becomes the essential actor inventing, defining and narrating a coherent self-identity, which is thus to be regarded as the product of a reflexive mental self-creation: [2]

"[...] [T]he narrative of self-identity has to be shaped, altered and reflexively sustained in relation to rapidly changing circumstances of social life, on a local and global scale. […] A reflexively ordered narrative of self-identity provides the means of giving coherence to the finite lifespan […]." (Giddens 1991: 215)

Methodologically, the character of individual biographical stories, including future life stories, bears several problems if used as a foundation of social science research. As Bourdieu (1998) argues, life stories present *biographic illusions*, imagining the life course as a consistent and coherent entity. They portray intentional

---

[2] Homi Bhabha and Anthony Giddens follow essentially different schools of thought in their conceptualizations of post-modern identity. Nevertheless both agree to acknowledge the multi-faceted and constructivist nature of self-identity, which is the aspect I relate to here.

moves and logical orders which reflect the personal rationality of life and the postulates about one's *raisons d'être*, while neglecting those elements of life that are arbitrary and shape the life course unpredictably and senselessly. Bourdieu's critique is important to this study, as it recalls the subjectivity and selectivity of life stories and cautions that conflicts and ambiguities will eventually not be postulated directly, but need to be revealed through analysis. While Bourdieu emphasizes the erratic character of real life courses, this study takes as a point of departure that a person's *raisons d'être* about life is still likely to impact his or her life course: as biographical research on women indicates, the personal self-perceptions, future visions and aspirations that shape one's *raisons d'être* formulate a frame of reference for the development of intentions to act in one way or another, that is for the future life script (Keddi 2008). They give implicit guidance to the individual decision-making in core questions of life.

The use of life stories as a data ground in this study is directed towards an exploration of this *raisons d'être* and its illusionary visions about a "happy future". The future life story is not expected to prescribe the future life course, but to translate individual and collective rationality and intentionality of life into guidelines for personal decision-making. Through the analysis of future life stories, the study aims at understanding individual and collective imaginations and rationalities of migration on the level of life plan and life script, rather than assessing the biographic correctness or feasibility of the life plan. Bourdieu's remark about contradictions of the life course being blurred in life stories has to be recognized as a general limitation of the data generated by future life stories as well. Notwithstanding this, research on future life scripts has shown that it is still possible to carve out inconsistencies and ambiguities through analysis (e.g. Keddi 2003).

### *Migration Intentions*

The early migration intentions of nursing graduates tackled in this study present an initiating factor in migration decision-making. This decision-making is firstly based upon concrete expectations, incorporating the person's awareness of problems and benefits involved in migration, and secondly upon the evaluation of their potential impact on the future life of an individual and/or a collective. De Jong (2000) found for migration from Thailand that expectancies of attaining valued goals in the future in other locations and low residential satisfactions with the current community were key determinants of intentions to move for men and women. Like individual life plans and life scripts, in particular immature, early expectations connected with migration are likely to be reshaped according to new information and life stage priorities and may not necessarily predict later migration decision-making - even more so as an abundance of external factors of migration decisions would have to be built into these expectations (see Table 1 p. 13).

Migration research and migration theory have been dealing with motivations and processes of migration decision-making as one of the central questions of the discipline, following different anthropological believes on human motivation, decision-making and action. The most commonly used "push-pull model" of migration, starts from the assumption that individuals are the main entity of life decision-making, following rational choices let by the aim to maximize their personal economic utility. Developed in the 1950$^{s}$ by W. Arthur Lewis, it originally explained migration as an economically reasoned reaction of an individual to unequal labour market opportunities between the place of residence and the respective destination. Throughout the following decades the model has been broadened to account for the influences of social capital and household decision-making. However its utilitarian paradigm of migration decision-making has hardly been challenged (Arango 2000, Boswell 2008). It presupposes that the reasons for migration decision-making were transparent, predictable and measurable, while complex structural contexts of migration decisions are neglected (Boswell 2008). The initially discussed influence of historical specifics, family and gender relations, traditions and networks of migration can hardly be taken into account under such a narrow umbrella, calling for a broader scheme of reference for this exploratory study.

The early phase of migration decision-making of the next generation of academic nurses in Malawi will instead be approached as an individual as well as collective phenomenon intertwining specific social and personal rationalities. The analytic focus on *social rationality* centres on the question how migration intentions are formed via culturally shaped conceptions of the collective, shared beliefs, norms and memories, which serve as symbolic ties. It considers the complex impact of observing others (Boswell 2008). The emphasis on *individual rationality* anchors the social dimension in the individual future perspectives, exploring how the individual remodels the collective rationalities of migration according to personal conditions and future aspirations.

### *Gender*

This study aims to be sensitive to gender-related differences in conditions and contexts of life planning and migration decision-making. Gender is considered as socially and historically shaped, but enacted on the level of personal agency:

> „[Gender is] a matrix of identities, behaviors, and power relationships that are constructed by the culture of a society in accordance with sex. [...] [W]hen people interact with each other, by adhering to [...] [the content of gender] or departing from it, they either reaffirm or change what is meant by gender, thus affecting social relationships at a particular time or in a particular setting. This means that gender is not immutable but also changes and, in this sense, is both socially constructed and reconstructed through time.“ (Boyd and Grieco 2003: n.p.)

On the individual level the agency of enacting (*doing*) and challenging (*undoing*) gender always presents as a paradox condition, as

> „the 'I' that I am finds itself at once constituted by norms and dependent on them but also endeavors to live in ways that maintain a critical and transformative relation to them.“ (Butler 2004: 3)

Mediating social images and relationships of gender, the contradictory day-to-day processes of mobilizing, negotiating and renegotiating gender affect concepts of life and future plans, as well as migration processes (Piper 2008). Social roles and rules of masculinity and femininity and how the students relate to these are therefore considered relevant to the analysis.

With regard to migration, gender has been discussed as an important pre-condition determining the likelihood, possibilities and circumstances of the mobility of women on three different levels, detailed in Table 2.

*Table 2. Factors Affecting Women's Preconditions for Migration*

| | |
|---|---|
| **Individual Level** | Age, birth order, race/ethnicity, urban/rural origins<br>Marital status, reproductive status,<br>Role and position in the family<br>Status e.g. educational, occupational skills and class position |
| **Family/ Household Level** | Size, age/sex composition, life-cycle stage and structure (nuclear, extended, etc.) of the family or household<br>Social status and class standing of the family<br>Relationships among family members (economic, emotional)<br>Gender relations and hierarchies of the household<br>Family attitudes towards migration |
| **Societal Level** | Structural characteristics, gender relations and hierarchies in society<br>Community norms, cultural values on forms (labour or family reunification) and constellations (alone or with family) of female migration |

Source: Adapted and amended from Boyd and Grieco 2003: n.p.

In the analysis of women nurses' migration intentions special regard will thus be attributed to their conditions in these three fields in the pre-migration stage. However, as gender concerns roles of masculinity as well as femininity, the study integrates male and female nursing students with migration prospects and approaches both groups under a gendered perspective.

## Data Collection

The data collection for this study was conducted in November and December 2010, within a three-month research stay in Lilongwe, the capital of Malawi. All students lived on the campus of the Kamuzu College of Nursing and were interviewed there. According to the official requirements to conduct medical research in Malawi, in the advent of the data collection authorization from the Kamuzu College of Nursing Research Chair and approval and advice from the Research and Ethics Commission of the College of Medicine (COMREC) in Blantyre were obtained. The consent form for the participation in this research was presented to the students in English and Chichewa on the campus board, together with the letter inviting them to participate. The students were given additional time in the beginning of a research sessions to read the form, clarify doubts and questions and sign it. Each of them obtained a copy signed by the researcher.

The initial phase of field research consisted in individually designed research workshops (WS), drawing on forms of focus group discussions described by Bloor (2001) and Fern (2001). Five workshops were conducted with an overall number of 39 participants aged between 21 and 25 years. The gender ratio of 30 female and 9 male participants reflects roughly the proportion of women and men in the student cohort graduating in 2010. The structure of the workshops allowed the participants to discuss issues in different settings, outlined in Table 3 (next page).

The workshop setting allowed exploring the nursing students' common images about nursing and migration and their perceptions of public opinions about nurse migration. It was furthermore chosen to promote a strong participation of the students in directing the course of discussion and give the researcher in the beginning a broad orientation about issues of concern that would be guiding the development of probe questions and guidelines for the following research phase of in-depth interviews. As I performed interviewing, moderating and data analysis, this proceeding was sought to expand my view from the beginning and thereby reduce the impact of

*Table 3. Structure of Research Workshops*

| | |
|---|---|
| **Introduction & personal focusing exercise** | Presentation of agenda, personal introduction; clarifying and signing of consent form<br>Personal questionnaire on individual future plans, attitudes towards migration, including selected personal features |
| **Small-group discussions** | Participants collected, discussed and wrote down their attitudes and experiences regarding the choice of nursing as a profession as well as motivations, experiences, advantages and disadvantages involved in nurse's migration in general. In WS 2 only topics were provided, in WS 1,3,5 focusing questions, in WS 4 controversial statements from the literature on nursing and migration. |
| **Whole-group discussions** | Main part of each WS (1-1,5h): students explained, commented, weighted and discussed the collected issues in dialogue with the researcher. Emerging new topics were added to the discussion. |
| **Closing** | Formal collection of feedback from students, informal dinner with the whole group |

my preconceived expectations on the agenda of discussion and the course of research. Students considering their migration projects a relatively confidential topic found in the introductory written activity an anonymous space to express. The following small-group activities encouraged the participants to raise controversial topics or take less accepted positions. At the same time, the individual and small-group activities worked as *focusing exercises* (Bloor 2001), deepening the students' attention to the topic.

During the whole-group discussion some controversial issues were discussed among the participants, however group dynamics sometimes limited the outcomes: questions aiming to provoke discussion of attitudes tended to lead into explanations about how this is generally perceived in Malawi or a repetition of opinions that had been agreed upon during the small-group discussions. Hierarchies in the groups, in particular male dominance, were too strong to make e.g. ranking exercises in the group feasible. The interaction among the students shifted often towards an exchange between group members and the moderator, making some of the conversations into group interviews rather than focus group discussions (Bloor 2001). The overall design of the workshops was accordingly rather adequate to give visibility to the groups' opinion then to generate insight via group interaction. However, unlike in an interview situation, the topics had been raised by the participants themselves and reflected the output of their initial discussions. The research workshops delivered the aspired collection and contextualisation of issues that students considered important. Their explanations were valuable to capture their approach towards the topic and the group setting was an effective icebreaker between students and researcher, advantaging the succeeding research.

Subsequent to the workshops, in-depth interviews were conducted with 7 female and 3 male nursing students. The students were selected according to theoretical criteria generated from the workshops and on the basis of the individual data from the initial questionnaire. The sample meant to present a broad spectrum of different constellations of attitudes and intentions regarding migration and nursing, varying future aspirations and personal characteristics including gender, family status and household composition.

The interviews followed a rough guideline of clustered topics and questions. Initially, the students were encouraged to talk about their broader biographic background with a focus set on the area of education. Afterwards near-future plans, overall life planning and their objectives in life were treated, with special regard to their plans and motivations to migrate. In the beginning of the conversations I used open, narrative questions which I were followed up with more directive and closed questions in later phases of the interview. In the interview situations open and broad questioning was sometimes answered relatively shortly or generating misunderstandings. [3] Rephrasing and in particular using examples for clarification narrowed or closed questions severally, leading to a

---

[3] I even recognized a personal tendency to avoid open questions where fearing misunderstandings.

more directive questioning than initially intended. While interviewees mostly found their way from a yes or no into self-revealing explanations that were useful as data, answers appearing to be biased by directive questioning were reflected cautiously and excluded from the analysis where it seemed indicated.

Besides the main research activities, talks and informal meetings were part of the field experience and are widely documented in a field-diary. A guideline-interview with a representative of the National Organisation of Nurses and Midwifes (NONM) and informal talks with KCN, NONM and NMCM representatives were held in order to gain a clearer background understanding of the perspective of nursing representatives on the situation of nurses and their motivations to migrate. Further "field activities" included a visit to two district hospitals and the participation in a review-meeting of students and their supervisors as well as, last but not least, the informal contact with the students throughout the whole period of data collection. A review of the NMCM migration register under the instructions of the registrar allowed gaining a clearer understanding of the existent data challenges there. These field activities were only very partially considered in the data analysis, but provided a valuable background understanding of nurses' and nursing students' living and working contexts and the social framing of the "nurse migration problem".

## Limitations

Beyond the already acknowledged methodical difficulties, general challenges throughout the study process concerned time constraints and a lack of adequate data sources and literature from Malawi. Unpublished or unavailable literature hindered for example the review of local scientists' perspectives on sociological questions of gender and migration. A time-consuming approval process and the students' time schedule reduced the time slots for organizing workshops and interviews to the minimum necessary.[4] The se-

[4] Though the research commissions were cooperative and the proposal prepared beforehand, the different requirements for an approval limited the time of data

quence of activities became however far too dense to allow for more than a rough analysis of main features on site, challenging the paradigm of grounded theory research to conduct data analysis hand in hand with further sampling and data collection. It was not possible to advance sufficiently with the data analysis to get to the point where full theoretical sampling could be assumed and a large part of the analysis had to be postponed to the aftermath of the research stay. A pronounced weakness is the lack of comparison between students with and without migration intentions: two nursing students (1 male/ 1 female) were selected for interviews, because their questionnaires had revealed negative attitudes and pre-decisions on migration. Selected to build up a comparison to those favouring migration, the interviews instead revealed that they were also considering leaving. In one case the deviant questionnaire response can be explained by a family conflict about migrating or staying; in the second case the reason could not be clarified.

Being part of a qualification process, this study was conducted by only one investigator, which challenges the important methodological suggestion that "*a grounded theorist need not work alone*" (Strauss and Corbin 1990b: 422). Conducting this research without a team was found to be demanding in terms of personal resources, especially during the moderation of research workshops and in the transcription phase. Teamwork is an acknowledged advantage in the process of coding to generate intersubjective perspectives on the data and improve the quality of the analysis (ibid.).[5] Though a careful and thorough data analysis and a critical review of findings were pursued, this lack is to be considered when drawing upon the results of this study. Working in a team with Malawian researchers would also have allowed to analyse more carefully the effects of researching as a white European the topic of

---

collection from three months to 6 weeks. As the students were furthermore performing clinical practices and examinations throughout the time of the field stay, the data-collection had effectively to be performed in one month.

[5] In this study the involvement of other researchers was reduced to the great help of Caroline, a Malawian student who crosschecked the transcripts in detail. Comments of several reviewers were worked upon thoroughly.

migration from an African country. According to findings of Aboderin (2007), interviewers with this positionality may e.g. provoke interviewees to understate the money-issue of migration in order to avoid the confrontation with the frequent negative stereotype among white Europeans that African nurses would just come for money.

On the conceptual level it has to be acknowledged that, working mainly upon individual life plans and scripts, the weight of the individual in the process of migration intention-building might be overestimated, as household or partners' influences and collective expectations are only taken into account to the extend to which they are highlighted by the individuals or openly considered with regard to the personal life plan. As decision-making structures, norms and roles within the household and wider social context are likely to constitute important influences on the young nurses' migration intentions and prospects, this constitutes an important limitation of the study.[6]

In view of the constraints mentioned above, the theoretical conceptualization of the findings became limited to segments of substantive theory on migration intentions in the life scripts and future plans of young nursing graduates. The exploratory concepts developed in the following chapters are meant to inform further qualitative and quantitative studies and theoretical reflections, which may formulate generalized theory on a broader empirical basis.

---

[6] Several family-specific questions regarding gender roles and the stake of the core family in life decision-making tended to be biased by the interviewers' questioning. This bias was widely taken into account when analysing the data, but leaves detailed insight into household and family decision-making to further research.

# IV. MIGRATION IN NURSES' FUTURE BIOGRAPHIES

The future ideas, life scripts and plans of nursing students that emerged from this study revealed a significant biographic importance of migration as a complex and encompassing *rite of passage* (see p. 15) with individually different shapes. Taking a overarching perspective on the interview data, I will firstly give a general idea of the common shapes of nursing students' biographic orientations, main traits of their self-identities and scripts of life, as well as a rough outline of commonalities of the encountered migration intentions. This panorama[1] is provided to clarify the broader contexts into which the individually specific life projects and migration intentions are built.

It is followed by detailed discussions on the role of migration in the different life projects that make up the students' future life plans. The sub-chapters are clustered along these life projects, which are outlined in Table 4. I approach these life projects as biographical orientations in the sense of *biographical horizons*, i.e. as durable guidance throughout particular life-periods or the overall life course (Keddi 2008; see p. 45). Each life project or biographic orientation is briefly described in the opening of the sub-chapter and explored in detailed with a view to individual biographic backgrounds and experiences and immanent scripts of life (i.e. values, motivations and self-identities), common social contexts (e.g. habitus, social discourses and gender patterns) and historical references (esp. (post)colonial *cultures of migration,* see p. 26). The professional project is tackled in the beginning and at more length than

[1] The findings presented here reflect the researchers' interpretation of the reported life plans, seen as a whole. Due to this, and in order to avoid duplications with the following detailed discussion, this sub-chapter is kept descriptive, without reference to data or literature. It may not stand for itself but requires the analytical fundament that is established in the course of the following discussion part.

the following life projects. This reflects the finding that the students emphasized the importance of educational and professional matters at the current point in their life, and accounts for the particularly complex interactions emerging between migration intentions and professional aspirations. It does however not mean to signal a lesser importance of the other life projects identified, acknowledging that the students' future biographies of migration may only be captured as an interrelationship of these projects.

Based on the detailed discussions of each life project and with reference to previous findings on nurse migration, the role of migration for each area of the envisaged future life is evaluated. Concluding the chapter, the findings are condensed towards an encompassing view on the students' future biographies of migration and reviewed regarding consequences for the migration, retention and return potential in this cohort of nursing students.

## General Life Scripts & Biographic Projects

Despite the high individual specificity of biographic priorities, common life themes and biographic projects could be identified based on the interviews and are roughly summarized in Table 4 to give a first orientation and structure to the following discussion. They reflect the students' embedding in a family, social and cultural context and reveal general ambitions to progress towards aspirational professional and private goals. With the exception of the partnership & parenthood project all interviewed students pursued these future plans. Their approaches varied regarding the main priorities and sequence of different life projects and the flexibility to adapt and follow alternative life plans e.g. regarding the question of educational upgrade and family-foundation.

*Table 4. Nursing Students' Biographic Orientations and Projects*

| | |
|---|---|
| **Professional Project** | (All) further education to at least master's level<br>(All) appreciative working-environments, satisfactory working results, responsibility on the job, opportunities for professional and career development<br>(Almost all) employment in leading positions of the health sector (Ministry, University, NGOs, managerial posts) |
| **Partnership & Parenthood Project** | (Most) get married, have children and live happily with them<br>[The others: happy single-life, independently or with family members] |
| **Family-related Project** | (All) good contact with families and receiving the family's respect<br>(All, different areas) contribute to the family's well-being (financially, caring for relatives, taking over responsibility and guidance for the younger) |
| **Social & Socioeconomic Project** | (All) reach a higher socioeconomic status<br>(Most) contribute to the development of the country, have own investments<br>(Most, directly or indirectly) become an important, socially appreciated person |
| **Personal Development Project** | (Most, to different degrees) pursue self-actualization, choose lifestyles, gain maturity<br>(Some) be economically independent, make individual life decisions |
| **Religious Orientation** | (All) let life be guided by ones God, live in accordance with religious ethics<br>(Several) provide service and religious guidance to others, develop spiritual maturity |

By far most students seemed to set the professional life project as first priority, the care for family members, marriage or motherhood were however often equally well-established milestones of the life plan. The envisaged sequence of milestones in their future lives varied particularly regarding the issue of partnership and children: one group aimed to pursue in the first place professional development and obtain economical independence, seen as a precondition of partnership, marriage and parenthood. The common scheme of another group was to get married and have a child before pursuing their professional plans. Where students had doubts if they would find the necessary chances to reach their goals, core challenges emerged in the areas of educational and professional development as well as gender empowerment.

### *Nurses' Concepts of Life and Self*

As exposed in the chapter on central concepts (see p. 43), this study assumes that students' explicit biographic orientations and plans are rooted in specific concepts of self and life that will be tackled in the following regarding main characteristics, congruencies and ambiguities. Insight on the nurses' professional plans and images of migration stem from the personal questionnaire, group-discussions and interviews alike, whereas the general future plans and visions tackled here go back exclusively to the in-depth interviews.

An overall positive outlook shaped the students' general approaches towards their future life. This is comprehensible in view of their current graduation marking the end of a college time that had embraced almost their entire social life since they had left their homes or boarding schools. The graduation presents a decisive starting point to set up and pursue more self-directed life plans. Beyond this situational factor, a general conviction that, at the end, a Christian God would direct their future life towards a foreseen path was perceived as a source of confidence to approach future with optimism and hope, and as a spiritual guidance through all future challenges.

Most students, men as well as women, expressed with clarity and assertiveness the will to follow an ambitious personal agenda for the coming years and highlighted the expectation to make fundamental choices either independently or in equal discussion with partners or family members. The latter aspect is distinctive in the Malawian context of youth empowerment, where a cultural principal of seniority interferes with decision-making entitlements and claims of youth (Mchakulu 2007; Mahowe 2005, NSO and ICF Macro 2010). Data on women with similar characteristics as the research population from the Malawi Demographic and Health Survey (MDHS) demonstrate that others, usually family members, often make the decisions on women's daily lives.

*Table 5. Malawian Women's Say in Specific Decisions by Background Characteristics 2010 (2004)*[2]

| **Background characteristic** | **Own health care** | **Large purchases** | **Daily purchases** | **Visits to family or relatives** | **All specific decisions**** | **Non of the specific decisions** |
|---|---|---|---|---|---|---|
| **Age 20-24** | (28)* 55 | (18) 24 | (31) 47 | (56) 65 | (13) 13 | (27) 25 |
| **Never married** | (17) | (9) | (10) | (21) | (8) | (72) |
| **(Secondary school or more)**<br>**More than secondary** | (32) 90 | (26) 71 | (34) 92 | (49) 94 | (20) 64 | (36) 1 |
| **Middle income** | (29) 52 | (20) 28 | (30) 49 | (55) 66 | (15) 17 | (24) 19 |

Sources: Mahowe 2005: 46 (MDHS 2004); NSO and ICF Macro 2011: 229 (MDHS 2010)

Mchakulu (2007) highlights that young people's self perceptions and behaviour partly reproduce the principle of elderly decision-making and favour dependence over independence, even if issues of particular importance to youth are concerned. In this context, it could have been expected that the students, in particular the women among them, would refer strongly to the family as unit of decision-making on future life issues. Instead, the nurses described biographic future visions grown out of the ambiguity between

[2] MDHS 2004: Percentage of women aged 15-49 who say that they alone or jointly have the final say in specific decisions, by background characteristics. In 2004 "all decisions" compiled additionally the decision whish food to cook today.
MDHS 2010: Percentage of currently married women aged 15-49 who usually make specific decisions either by themselves or jointly with their husband, by background characteristics.

affirmation of age- or gender-related decision-making constraints, and empowerment aspirations and strategies - leaning confidently towards individual decision making claims. Female as well as male participants stated to negotiate their decisions assertively with family members and colleagues, and several disclosed an individually focused life planning scheme in the sense that the realization of personal goals and priorities was formulated as ultimate end of decision-making in life. The general claim for individual *ownership* in decision-making constitutes a common angle of the young nurses' life scripts and acts as an impulse towards emancipative lifestyles, repercussive in different areas of the individual life plans. *Ownership* is used here in a non-material sense as a signifier for a personal identification with decisions and actions, strengthening the feeling of involvement and participation. It means to express the students' attitude of having the right to establish and pursue personal life plans according to their goals, values and self-identities as well as to take biographic decisions in their own name.

Ambitious goals and high expectations compared to their current situation emerged as a second common characteristic of the students' life scripts and self-perceptions: to "*be hard working*", "*assertive*", "*score best*" and "*aim high in life*"[3] were frequent, biographically sustained self-attributions, designing a strategy of action that could be summarized as 'If you are given a chance in life, take it and make the very best out of it, dedicating it hard work, optimistic believe and confidence to make the difference. Then you will find possibilities to reach far and be successful'.

Remarkably high self-expectations became tangible in many areas of the envisaged future, whether regarding ones professional projects, self-development and partnership, spirituality or social commitment and moral backbone. They shape a *character of ambition* that can be linked to the students' academic habitus, revealing an elite self-identity and reflecting common public expectations towards members of the highly educated class. It manifests in firm commitments to lead a life according to the values of ones God,

[3] These expressions were extracted and coded from the interview transcripts as repetitively mentioned core self-attributes.

contribute extraordinarily to the development of ones country, profession and the status of the beloved ones and to stand up for ones personal rights as women, nurses etc. Incorporating ambition, assertiveness and commitment, the nurses portray an understanding of *ownership* of their future life that aims at the realization of one's life goals in accordance with individual and collective interests alike.

Bringing together the students' concepts of self and life, Table 6 (next page) names 'character' types, which show congruencies between their self-identities, scripts of life and biographic future priorities. These 'characters' are abstract categories disconnected from the individual cases. They mean to sketch out different priorities guiding the individual biographic outlooks and shaping diverging sub-contexts of the individual migration intentions. The *Care-Giver* character, evoking an idealized image of nursing, guides towards an emphasis on the collective embeddedness of the life course, in a sense of being socially integrated and recognized, embedding ones' decisions into the context of family needs and orienting the life-course towards collective aims (e.g. family solidarity, family formation) and stable conditions. The *Nobile* character derives from the use of the term by Bourdieu (1986: 53), who attributes it to a publicly known subgroup of persons, speaking on behalf of and exercising authority in the name of a whole group. It is used here to refer to those degree nurses whose social and professional aspirations are directed by a desire to distinguish themselves from what they perceive to be an ordinary Malawian nurse - attempting to make a change in the profession and aiming towards political and other leadership positions, trying not to become an "*average person*" (Interview P5M, 7), but a well recognized citizen of the Malawian society e.g. making huge investments into charity and contributing to the country's development.

*Table 6. Cluster of Biographic Orientations, Self-identities and Life Scripts*

| Character | Biographic Priorities | Self-Identity Patterns | Life Script Priorities | Guiding Biographic Principles |
|---|---|---|---|---|
| **The Care-Giver** | Settlement | Altruistic | Spiritual peace/maturity | Status stability |
| | Well-off family | Family-related | Family harmony | Value stability |
| | Economic & job security<br>*Embeddedness* | Oriented tow. the collective | Collective well-being | Collective happiness |
| | Moral firmness<br>Religious activity | Conservative | Traditional values | |
| **The Nobile** | Titles | Elitist | Social status | Status mobility |
| | Leadership positions | Controlling | Self-affirmation | Prestige |
| | Appreciative job environment | Power-seeking | Social & professional power | Progress |
| | High well-being<br>Charity Investment | Moralist<br>'"Patriotic" | National development | Leave footprints |
| **The Reformer** | Acad./ prof. development | Academic | Self-actualisation | Excellence |
| | International exposure | Innovative | Social innovation | Innovation |
| | Pers. & econ. independence | Individualist | Cultural change | Emancipation |
| | Modern lifestyle | Modern | Lifestyle choice | Independence |
| | Social innovation | Emancipated | Self-determination | Individual happiness |

### *Ambiguities of the Life Script*

In the individual future biographies, the characters outlined in Table 6 overlap, interact and compete, often establishing an ambiguous future outlook into which migration intentions are positioned. One prominent area of ambiguity emerging on the level of life script and life plan regards individual self-determination on one side, compliance towards responsibilities and predefined roles in family and society on the other side. This tension reflects a social ambivalence between a strong local culture of family solidarity and collective orientation, and the influence of a global context of social modernization that emphasizes individual choice and decision-making throughout the life course and in the narrative of self-identity. As Giddens (1991) showed for other contexts, the young generation of Malawian nurses perceives binding orders of traditional roles as negotiable in reference to a global social space, associated with freedom of lifestyle choices and diversity in the personal and public sphere. The emerging tension shapes the students' projects of migration and return, their motivations to leave respectively return, and the character of the envisaged lifetime abroad.

A second ambiguity evolves between aspirations to secure socioeconomic stability for oneself and members of the family, and an agenda of social and professional progress and innovation, relating to the character of ambition. The students' concrete life plans integrate these poles in different ways: sequencing the imagined life course into times for mobility and times for stability, envisioning uncommon forms of settlement or relationship, or drafting different life projects in opposite ways. Aspirations towards the pole of personal, professional, and social mobility built a main motivator to migrate, while they are commonly embedded into larger life concepts oriented towards stable socioeconomic conditions, securing a reliably good quality of life allowing to settle and found a family.

A third ambiguity in the students' life plans directly regards migration, establishing between the aspirations towards a life stage abroad and the ethical valuing of '*making one's contribution*' in

Malawi. This ambiguity reflects the body of social images about the benefits of nurse migration on the one hand, a social expectation to be successful in and for Malawi on the other hand. These contradicting aspirations are negotiated by means of different legitimizing argumentations within the professional, personal and religious life projects and become concrete in the most commonly envisaged plan to migrate temporarily. The findings point out that existing ethic objections against migration have to be counterbalanced with the expected individual and social benefits.

### *Migration in the Life Plan*

As a general observation, migration owns a preponderant position in the study participants' future biographies. Migration prospects enter the individual life plans of most interviewees as an important opportunity to access the envisaged level of education, to develop their life projects and facilitate compatibility between them, as well as to beware them from failure and socioeconomic insecurity in Malawi. The idea of *greener pastures abroad* is brought up recurrently, as in many studies on migration intentions of African health workers (e.g. Awases et al. 2004; Grigulis 2010; Dovlo 2003). It can be regarded as a symbol signifying the trend among Malawian nurses to imagine and seek migration as a promising means towards a not further determined better life. More concretely, many nurses assume that migratory experience would provide them, on the long track, with valuable professional, social and personal resources to pursue different aspirations, ranging from economic well-being and social status to self-determination and lifestyle choice. The personal questionnaire, a card survey and rating of priorities regarding migration in WS 5 delivered first insights into personal migration intentions. A clearer picture shaped in the interviews, when migration prospects were discussed in detail in the context of each student's wider life planning.

It is the access to higher education that emerges as the most essential expected benefit and accordingly as the main motivation to leave: All students involved in this study were seeking to improve their academic education and almost all considered or favoured the option to go abroad for their master studies, notwithstanding the existence of ethic objections against migration. Students who favoured the idea of a stay abroad expected that the realization of their overall life goals would require a more favourable environment of personal, professional and social development than accessible in Malawi. Students whose expectations were in turn captured by fears to suffer socially, personally or spiritually, described migration as a last option, needed to extend the educational and professional capacities that would be needed to attain their life goals in a later future in Malawi. Their fears were connected with the distance to family members, racist discrimination and violence as well as challenges related to language and access to accommodation. Though several dangers of migration in the psychosocial field such as family break-up, loss of cultural relatedness and social bonds, as well as confrontation with public displeasure were foreseen, they were often projected exclusively to those who would not return to settle.

At the same time, the common view that those succeeding abroad would come back skilled, changed, rich and modernized was associated with the expectation of high social appreciation for those who would return (ibid.). Annex Table 1 gives an overview on the students' common views on the positive and negative aspects of Malawian nurses' migration from different perspectives.

Most students confirmed a strong inclination towards temporary migration of two to five years: while a number of graduates expressed readiness to take the chances of migration as a means to a comfortable and independent life abroad, most students approached migration as a way to improve their preconditions for success and a good life in Malawi. Where students were open or even favouring to spend their future life outside Malawi, satisfaction of their professional, family and individual aspirations was projected into the idea of a life abroad. With reference to these general concepts of self, life and migration, the following discussion of the nursing graduates' biographic projects analyses and theoretically contextualizes the specific functions of migration in different areas of the life plan.

## The Professional Project

The main features of the students' professional life projects can be summarized as follows: at the time of data collection all students were finishing their final examinations and waiting for a call by the public health service to place them in different governmental hospitals all over the country, where they were supposed to deliver their years of obligatory duty.[4] The majority of students accepted to do two years of obligatory bedside service before progressing with their career, valuing the working experience and salary to pay off debt and obtain the qualifications to apply for further education. The majority had integrated bedside nursing into their life plan as an initial stage of a professional career progressing towards higher academic titles and managerial or political positions in nursing or other fields of the health sector. Despite that, a few students expressed consent or desire to do bedside or community nursing in the long run. For them, the prospect to work in the ward beyond the time of obligatory service was however usually connected with fears of a professional and personal stagnation that could endanger educational progress and professional development - central drivers of their future vision and life script. All 39 students revealed a plan to go on with their studies up to the master level, 9 students even aimed to continue up to a PHD. The professional migration intentions referred usually to 2-5 years stays dedicated to pursue a master degree abroad. They related mostly to the time after the envisaged years of obligatory duty; only one interviewee was already actively trying to find a scholarship abroad.

The essential role of migration in most professional life projects emerges foremost from a biographic focus on further education and professional career. Secondly it results from an evaluation of local against global conditions to realize professional plans and coordinate them with other life projects. The discussion in this chapter departs from the perceived vulnerability of the professional

---

[4] According to Tambulasi and Chasukwa (2015), the current bonding scheme provides for 5 years of obligatory service. The nurses however constantly referred to two years.

project in the Malawian occupational context. From there, the understanding of the professional motivations to migrate is broadened, integrating the biographic importance of educational, social, ethic and gender aspects of the professional self-identity into the picture. The students' common, enthusiastic imagination about migration-to-study is explored regarding inherent references to historically shaped and transnationally enacted images of nurse migration, as well as ideas about membership of a mobile, global academic elite. Going beyond general scripts of professional identity and migration, gender differences are highlighted as markers of the students' professional identity and biographic outlook as nurses, with consequences for the expected impacts of migration on the professional life project.

### *The Vulnerability of the Professional Project*

At the roots of the migration intentions in the students' professional life projects lies a negative evaluation of their chances to develop professionally within the occupational environment of nurses in Malawi. This is coupled with apprehensions that the local occupational reality would provoke failure of the professional project on different levels. A condensed compilation of the graduates' professional ambitions, frustrations and individual consequences is provided in Table 7 (see p. 70). It reveals how concrete working conditions, hospital hierarchies and socio-political structures of the Malawian health system are perceived to translate into barriers to professional satisfaction, status and career development, and into core drivers of the students' professional life projects.

Frustrating working conditions in the hospital regard foremost personal recognition, safety from infection, quality of care/ satisfying outcomes, under-staffing and payment, and disclose in the students' professional plans as a push factor towards managerial positions and alternative work settings (e.g. community work and advocacy). These frustrations reflect closely the occupational challenges documented in the literature on nurses in Malawi's public health system (Muula and Maseko 2006; Manafa et al. 2009; Durevall and Mussa 2010; DFID 2010).

*Table 7. Occupational Aspirations, Constraints and Individual Reaction*

| Level | Working Conditions in Hospitals | Hospital Hierarchies | Socio-Political Structures |
|---|---|---|---|
| Aspirations | Apply qualifications & deliver good nursing care | Responsibility on the job | Public Recognition for ones effort and service, Representation of Nurses Affairs |
| | Satisfactory caring results for patients, public & themselves | Influential positions (e.g. ward in-charge)/ power to shape services and conditions | Stable contract and payment conditions |
| | Having a long and healthy professional life | Professional recognition as highly-qualified nurse, Appreciative staff team, possibilities of capacity development on the job | Access to further education within the next 5 years |
| Constraints | Lack of resources & staff, settings of improvisation, low quality care | Fixed hospital hierarchies structured by years of duty | Feeling that the political level represents only patients', not nurses' affairs |
| | Lack of qualification and commitment of colleagues, unfortunate staff allocation, communication and management failures | Seniority principle, discrepancies between their level of education and their position (e.g. being supervised and judged by diploma holders) | Insecurity of first working-placements, unexpected reduction of payment till NMCM license is obtained (student contract) |
| | Low hygiene standards and awareness | Disrespecting, absent are incompetent supervisors, leaving young nurses alone with problems | Long waiting lists for midwifery course, high competition for master's in Malawi, long waiting lists for government-sponsored master's places |

| Level | Working Conditions in Hospitals | Hospital Hierarchies | Socio-Political Structures |
|---|---|---|---|
| Resulting Problems | Limited possibilities to practice the quality care they were taught to deliver | No participation in management decisions; little responsibility | Economic precariousness |
| | Destruction of the fruits of work and effort, powerlessness against curing failures and patients' death | Slow upward-mobility into higher positions, no performance-based upgrades | Unsettledness of future plans |
| | Facing negative public reputation of nurses, being unsatisfied with the results of one's work, High infection risks and fear of infection | Poor access to trainings on the job, reduced motivation to perform well, unfortunate learning-conditions at the bedside | Frustration of ambitious life plans |
| Individual Consequences | Learning and practising good nursing abroad | Negotiation of employment conditions | Upgrade in education (Master) to enter positions in the Ministry in order to make a political change for nurses, Looking for opportunities abroad and in the private sector |
| | Upgrade in education (Master) to enter managerial and political positions and promote changes | Obtainment of a master's degree to insure fast upgrading into influential positions | |
| | Focus on community nursing and health advocacy/awareness work outside the hospital, Focus on Psychiatric nursing (less infection risk), NGO work | Leaving the hospital setting into managerial or NGO settings | |

The young nurses' perspectives on their working reality in Malawi are formed by their experiences during several months of clinical practices in different government hospitals, as well as their contacts with government health institutions. In their clinical practices they encountered power relations informed by seniority and favouritism, associating their young age with greenness, denying to them responsibilities and entitlements to suggest adjustments. The low entitlements of the young generation of nurses may be seen here as a reflection of the already tackled low decision-making authority of Malawian youth more generally.

"[…] [the problem] is that like here in Malawi, the nursing profession - you would see that most of the people - when you are trying to make maybe a change in something - they would say: you are very young. What do you want to do, want to say? Like those veterans who have been working maybe for more than 20 years, 30 years - frankly speaking they discourage us... You would see that maybe the District Nursing Officer would say: we are having this workshop - of which I believe, attending the workshop, it's also part of professional development, because you went there and you gained some new knowledge - they would say: Ah, should we take this one or this one? This one is so young; she has just come this year, let her be working in the ward." (Interview P2F: 11)

Also with regard to the nursing management, the study participants complained about the association of entitlement with seniority and the problem of arbitrariness of nursing managers as well as governmental nursing institutions. E.g. in workshop 1 and 4 students complained about young qualified staff's difficulties to enhance changes and speak up for their own interests, as they would be supposed to serve in the least attractive areas before being given these right. Concrete issues the students raised against the nursing management concerned that the salaries for graduates were cut down to the amount of a student allowance till the license of the NMCM would be obtained, and that several days after the final examinations students had not yet received their work placements, though they should have been informed two weeks earlier. These changes unsettled students who had planned and/or necessitated to generate income immediately after their studies. Research by

Tambulasi and Chasukwa (2011) and Muula and Maseko (2006) support the students' perception about unclear career paths and sluggish promotional processes. The authors highlight in particular the absence of a Health Service Commission in charge of health workers' promotion, and the institutional discrimination of degree nurses against clinical officers in awarding leading functions (see p. 33-34).

Though in general the students showed high appreciation for their lecturers, many alluded to a lack of encouraging supervision practices in college and clinical experiences and perceived certain information and decision-making practices as an affront towards their learning interests and rights. The study participants complaint in this regard that the college administration obliged them to work while writing their research papers, though they had been promised two weeks off. Furthermore the student representatives had objected and successfully battled against the attempt of the college administration to channel them into placements for clinical practices without considering their priorities. A perceived lack of acknowledgement for their effort and their status as learners became even more tangible concerning supervision in the work place:

> "But you go to work, you work, you work and at the end someone comes and he shouts at you: Hey hey hey, why did you do that? This ahead really demotivates you. But you should see, you should feel, when some other people, someone who looks at us, they should try to appreciate that this is what we are doing and we are doing good. And some areas of improvement - these are the areas that you can improve. That motivates me." (Interview P32F: 18)

In the students' eyes, these conditions limit their possibilities as highly qualified and ambitious junior staff to participate in decision-making and management, to apply and improve their knowledge and capacity, and to be called into higher and more rewarding positions. In consequence, they impede that the young graduates' educational status after four years of academic training would translate into a higher occupational status that could satisfy their professional ambitions. While the concrete roots of the named problems can be located in the nursing hierarchy, they appear as reflections of broader social issues: as Buchmann (1998 on the USA) has accentuated, the challenge to translate educational capital into occupational status constitutes a core challenge and aspiration in young people's life-course planning within modern societies. While the social and labour market contexts of the USA and Malawi as well as the reasons for occupational status insecurity differ considerably, both contexts share this core challenge and its importance to the professional life-course planning of educated youth.

Though the young nursing students approach their professional environment with frustration in the first place, the prospect of changes constitutes a motivating factor. Several students contest the encountered conditions in Malawi with a strong ambition to "*make some change in caring for people*" (Quest. P2F), in political and structural grievances regarding nursing, as well as in the quality of care at the bedside. The idea to make a change in the nursing profession, referring to caring for people, nursing management and politics, was recurrent in several interviews and workshops (e.g. WS1, Interview P2F, Interview P25).[1] Their visions of change build on their academic training knowledge about health care problems in Malawi. Aspirations to make a contribution to improve the practice and status of nursing in Malawi are expressed with an attitude of protest as well as commitment towards the professional mission of nursing, in particular tangible among female students.

This attitude reveals most clearly in the interview and discussion statements of P25, a female nurse, who evaluates her moral self-expectation to care against the envisaged obstacles to encourage changes to the conditions of nursing and her major concern of professional development. She strongly rejects to work under the given circumstances in Malawian hospitals, which she regards as degrading to nurses and patients. Emphasizing that for her the political effort to change these is a condition for working in Malawi, she affirms her readiness to leave the country otherwise. At the same time, she expresses a strong vocation to deliver nursing care from the heart and defined ideas about the contribution she

[1] Where the expression is repeated in the following, it alludes to the named interviews.

plans to make to change nursing in Malawi: preventing nutritional health issues as a community nurse, she hopes to counteract the perceived problem that patients coming to the hospital are often already too ill to be cured (Interview P25; WS 4).

### *The Biographic Importance of Education*

Biographically formed self-perceptions deliver an important background to understand the students' priority on education, which in the Malawian context of academics (in nursing and beyond) associates with a susceptibility to go abroad.[2]

The biographic stories collected reveal education as a fundamental life script element. Most interviewed students settle their decision to go far with education in their early childhood or, less often, in secondary school age, encouraged and supported by motivating attitudes towards education in their social environment, usually by parents, siblings or extended family members or – in substitute – by neighbours, teachers or friends. Nine out of ten interviewees subsequently acknowledge family's, neighbour's, teacher's encouragement and assistance as an essential factor in their schooling careers. Solely one male interviewee describes that his family was little inclined to education and attributed his schooling success to good leaning results and personal interest in school. Beyond psychological encouragement, several interviewees report that their father's intervention had been necessary to open the chance to enter a good secondary school, as by examination performance they had only been selected to low-quality Community Day Secondary Schools.

These findings point to family values and expectations, as well as family solidarity as essential driving forces towards educational attainment of most nursing students. Even where parents count with no or minor educational attainment, the students' family and social backgrounds embody high levels of cultural capital in their habitus, treating schooling as a priority and being ready to invest in it while educating the children to be hard-working at school. In particular among students' fathers, continued education and late

---

[2] See Chapter Malawian (Nurses') History of Migration, p. 26-29.

entry into tertiary education are common, so that many students observed adult education at home as a good choice in life and were thankful that they were given the chance of tertiary education early in their life-courses already. Family encouragement to pursue education, and parents' use of higher education to improve the situation of the family during students' childhood time, establish education as an essential value and rewarding resource to secure well-being and reputation. Role-models' and parents' arguments to reach high in education range from obtaining higher income for the family, increasing chances to find a well-situated husband and improve ones social status, to the furthering of personal intellectual and career ambitions – arguments which transmit a broad value of education for a successful future also beyond the professional life project.

Previous studies (Grigulis 2010) as well as impressions from this study suggest that the socioeconomic background of Malawian nursing graduates is relatively heterogeneous, including also students from poor families. In low-income contexts, the valuing and support of education in the family appears to have particularly high importance. As also found by Jamison and Lockheed (1985) regarding children's schooling in Nepal, beyond the socioeconomic situation the attitudes towards education in the family reveal as decisive for students educational attainment. In our context, even where family members' encouragement on schooling was not connected with own educational attainment, the students reported they had been raised to value education as a core biographic resource.

It is notable that all students talk about (in particular fathers' and brothers') “encouragement”, but never about pressure. This indicates that the young nurses follow an intergenerational principal and biographic guideline to value educational success and uphold a self-perception as hard-working person. In line with this interpretation, several individual stories of students[3] point to their high personal commitment for education, even in episodes of economic hardship, when family encouragement was unavailable, or

[3] E.g. Interviews P5M, P25F and P2F

where low performance and frustrations of professional prospects affected their success. The students' general character of ambition reveals most clearly with regard to this educational and professional life project and is to be evaluated as an essential personal quality to promote a successful professional future.

According to Bourdieu (1986), the family represents the core institution for the transmission and embodiment of cultural capital, defined as accumulated labour that, in embodied form (as disposition), objectified form (as cultural good) or institutionalized form (as socially objectified disposition), creates cultural capacities to generate further cultural capital and translate it into profits on the level of social and economic status (Bourdieu 1986). In consequence, the presence of high appreciation and support of education in the students' families and social environment can be regarded as a privileging condition to accumulate the cultural capital of education from early childhood on. The individual training performance and commitment towards extraordinary success at school, as well as a high awareness of the usefulness of this resource to expand economic as well as social power indicate the embodiment of educational capital at a within the Malawian context distinguishing level, bearing a *symbolic profit of distinction* in the sense of Bourdieu:

„[…] the specifically symbolic logic of distinction additionally secures material and symbolic profits for the possessors of a large cultural capital: any given cultural competence (e.g., being able to read in a world of illiterates) derives a scarcity value from its position in the distribution of cultural capital and yields profits of distinction for its owner." (Bourdieu 1986: 245)

The young nurses' biographical awareness of education as a capital constitutes an important determination of future (cultural) capital acquisition (Bourdieu 1986) and can be regarded as essential for their strategy to pursue their professional life project by being hard-working and aiming towards distinguishingly high levels of education.

The nursing profession has commonly been associated with job security and stable income, i.e. a modest but settled economic situation (see Table 8, p. 87). Furthermore it had received a symbolic social prestige from the positive connotation of nursing with high skills and a Christian vocation to care (Grigulis 2010). The relatively recent introduction of academic training for Malawian nurses positions the young nursing graduates in-between a context of professional ideology honouring altruism and decent mediocrity, and an academics' context requiring self-promotion as well as ambition towards high socioeconomic status and socially sanctioned *nobility*.

"What happens here is: you find that you have upgraded, you have gone high with your studies, you are a nurse. Then you are called into managerial positions". (Interview P25F: 20)

From a broader societal perspective and considering the exclusivity of education in Malawi (see p. 22-24), the privileged status of a graduate engenders a body of public images that engrave high expectations to academic nurses' *public life course*, such as the attainment of personal success, social status and well-being of oneself and family members (including e.g. health care, protection of the pension-age life standard, financial, housing and education needs of siblings' families). While also lower cadres of nurses may find themselves in a struggle for the appreciated upgrading prospects in nursing (Manafa et al. 2009), the public view on the highly-skilled young nurses and their social contexts of reference tend to be associated with higher career expectations compared to general Malawian nurses' public life course frame.

Frustrated career expectations thus exacerbate into a status conflict for academically trained nurse at the point of occupational orientation and life planning, where low occupational career potentials on the Malawian government-nurses' labour market stand against their ambitious professional goals and the social expectations towards them as young academics and junior professionals of Malawi's educated elite. Resulting from the multileveled barriers to their professional development, the students express fears that a career 'from the scratch' of bedside nursing would not allow them to develop towards a professional status that could satisfy their status aspirations after four years of academic training considering positions and responsibilities in the occupational hierarchy, income and public recognition as an important person. Further academic qualification, assumedly enhancing opportunities of promotion and access to positions on ministerial level, is taken as the most viable exit-strategy towards new development potentials (see Table 7: *Individual consequences*, p. 70), pointing to the students' academic self-identities prioritizing educational titles and skill development over fast financial security. Where students see the health NGO sector in Malawi as an alternative, it tends to appear in the second place or as an opportunity for later years. While employment in NGOs or IOs in Malawi is attractive due to high salaries, its recognized weakness concerns the lack of opportunities for local stuff to develop professionally and access further education (RoM et al. 2007). The students show an awareness of this situation in their planning, as they prefer the government system as employer throughout the first years, while NGO employment is considered a tempting step to improve ones income in later years of the professional project. Interestingly, difficulties of a return from abroad into the Malawian social and working environment were hardly considered as challenges connected with a temporary migration plan to pursue ones professional project: only one workshop group mentioned difficulties to return into the Malawian working environment as one long-term challenge of migration, however not a priority issue.

### *Nursing as a Career Compromise*

The process of career choice-making shads some further light on the shared priority of the students on education and their strategy of action to obtain professional goals. All students had reached high MSCE results at the end of secondary school and were decided to head towards tertiary education. However, the nursing profession was not what most participants were initially striving for: by far the majority of the participating female students had applied in the first place (and often also in the second and third place), for other careers, ranging from Agricultural Engineering and Business Administration over Law, Political Sciences and

Media for Rural Development to General Medicine. Several students indicated that the majority of their classmates (beyond those participating in the study) had also been selected into nursing, though their choices had been in other study-areas, pointing to a general practice of channelling students into nursing. Where female students did not vote to do a degree in nursing they were usually selected into the career by the University of Malawi, which had to fill more study places in nursing in recent years. It is likely that the increased number of study places in BSc Nursing, compared to the capacities of other degree programmes, led to a misbalance between demand and supply, provoking a need to channel applicants of other programmes into the nursing career.[4]

Most female nursing students accordingly faced an early deflection of their envisaged professional future, implying the necessity to abandon their original professional interest for an acceptable trade-off and to develop motivation and ambition for nursing as a profession connected with particular personal challenges. To enter an UNIMA required therefore not only excellent performance at school, but also the readiness to make a fundamental compromise.

“Participant P25F: I never thought of becoming a nurse, I was someone who was so afraid of seeing patients, even I would cry if someone is sick at home I would not go closer to them.

Researcher: Oh, so you had a hard time.

Participant P25F: But now everyone tells me to say: hey, you are very good in the clinic, but I never liked even visiting people in the hospital: if my mum or dad takes me to the hospital to see a patient I would stay or sit outside, I would never go in. Oh, but now I have grown to do best.

Researcher: It must have been very hard though...

Participant P25F: Very, ya, even the first day I came here, it was very

[4] The training capacities in nursing had been raised quickly in an initiative by the Malawian Ministry of Health and several development partners to address the country’s nurse shortage. In order to enter the study programme students still had to pass an examination particularly focusing questions regarding motivations and ethics of nursing.

difficult for me when they took us for orientation. It was bad, very very difficult. But then little by little I developed it." (Interview P25F: 5)

While several female students confessed that they perceived and accepted their selection into nursing as a prophecy by their God, they made at the same time a decision against their original vocation to maintain educational career prospects. The admission into the nursing programme accordingly classifies as a religious call and an open door towards a professional career based on academic qualification.

Most male students had aimed to become Medical Doctors but failed in the entrance examinations of the College of Medicine. They chose nursing following rumours that a switch from the nurses' to the physicians' study programme would easily be possible (WS 1; WS 2). These rumours refer back to what nurses had told them when holding promotion talks in secondary schools and confirm the social influence on the students' status-related career decisions. The students frequently acknowledged that the advice of family members, friends and acquaintances as well as public images and rumours about nursing (Table 8, next page) had shaped their decision to accept the profession. Promotion talks informed students with no initial motivation for the profession about the external status-related benefits of the nursing profession: in particular they highlighted opportunities of career advancement, eventually connected with migration opportunities, and the security of immediate employment after studies, advocating for a career compromise that would be compatible with young school-leavers social status aspirations. Only one student (WS2, P12F) reported that her parents had convinced her to choose nursing instead of law because of her kindness, suggesting a latent influence of gender images as well.

*Table 8. Advisors' Arguments to Join the Nursing Profession*

| **Employment Status** | **Educational Status** | **Social Status** | **Personal Development** | **Family Expectations** |
|---|---|---|---|---|
| Job-security<br>Fast employment<br>Comparatively high payment | Chances to upgrade in education | Public recognition of nurses<br>Attention to the white uniform<br>Stable financial situation | Development of traits of kindness | Qualification to care for relatives |
| | Migration prospects | | | |

The students' compromise values status over vocational interests and stands in accordance with the psychological observation of Gottfredson (1981), who argues that the area of vocational interest only gains influence in career compromise-making where sex-type and prestige level are minimally acceptable (i.e. the occupation is within a person's *social space*) (Gottfredson 2005). The theory of Gottfredson on professional decision-making argues that career decisions are usually taken in reference to expected professional status, but not always aim towards the highest possible status because the individual's *social space* tends to regulate his or her aspirations: Accordingly, vocational compromise follows the individual's self-positioning in a *social space*, excluding professions whose sex type, prestige level or difficulty are evaluated as inappropriate in the person's social reference group and from its social vantage point. According to Gottfredson, only within this framework occupational options are later prioritised by the expected personal fulfilment and compatibility with personal characters (ibid.). In turn, people only look outside their *social space* when they see no accessible options within it, pushing their tolerable prestige level boundary further out than they do with their tolerable sex-type boundary (Gottfredson 1981). Not to accept the University's offer to study nursing would have meant to risk the social status and appreciation connected with tertiary education at the (locally prestigious) University of Malawi (UNIMA), and eventually loose the access to tertiary education at all.

"[...] the problem is about the chances that one has here in Malawi. When an opportunity presents itself to pursue higher education, personal education, you just take it because it presented itself (others laugh agreeing), because we know: it's an opportunity for you and you will loose it! Because maybe, many think that, comparing to other countries, whereby when you want to do something, you really have the choice to do something, you really do that thing, you do it. Maybe in the position we are given, we have been forced into the profession because we had no other option. So it's different here: when you have been selected to do personal education, you just take the chance." (WS 1, P4F: 3)

That the young nurses commonly subordinated their vocational interest to the chance to obtain educational status constitutes also a legacy of educational success at the roots of their professional identity, perpetuating the importance of academic progress into future. Relating the students' biographic experience of education to their individual life plans, with Gottfredson it may be argued that they develop their professional identity and aspiration in the frame of an elite *social space* of reference that demands a prestigious level of education. Being a graduate was frequently used as self-attribute and proof of the personal ability to pursue higher goals in education and in life, which additionally highlights the deep entanglement of personal and professional identity.

Furthermore, many students described that their extraordinary educational success had earned them an important role-model position, i.e. a status improvement, in their family[5] and beyond. The strong academic focus of the peer group of nursing graduates and the broader social reference group of Malawian academics establishes high educational attainment as the essential social element of common professional identity, necessary to pursue social membership and opportunities to develop social and socioeconomic capital in the sense of Bourdieu (1986). As will be further explored

[5] Even if older siblings had also managed to enter tertiary education, their success to have entered the public university UNIMA was mostly exclusive in the family.

in the chapter on going global and turning homewards (see p. 139-46), this elite academic *social space* is to be understood as a transnational rather than a local space, as the group shares a habitus of global social membership through education.

The deviant case of a woman who had chosen nursing independently as her first career option, against her family's advice to become a physician, strengthens these findings. Her story highlights the importance of migration in a context where bedside nursing is the professional prospect, and religious motivations to serve God via nursing care dominates the professional future vision: her migration intention clearly restricts to the opportunity of further academic education in psychiatric nursing, a speciality inaccessible in Malawi and sought to promote her skills in an area of nursing with low infection risks and highly needy patients. Her migration intentions remain subordinated to religious obligations and the imperative to care for needy family members, putting freedom of worship in the country of destination as a condition and restricting migration to other African countries. While migration inscribes into her professional vision to serve as highly skilled nurse in Malawi's public system, the academic self-identity of aiming towards higher education continues to be the professional driver to leave:

> "So it's like you get developed by and by professionally, as you are working in the district or where ever they have posted you. But (sighing) still that wouldn't be enough; we would still want to do something a little bit higher." (Interview P31F: 16)

The case highlights that even degree nurses who did not choose nursing as a mere career compromise count with an academic professional self-identity and social identity, demanding to seek further educational and skill progress. This questions whether students selecting the career independently would be less touched by the dynamics of education, career and migration, as it strengthens the general finding that the nursing students share biographies focusing educational attainment as mayor resource for a successful professional and personal future.

According to Manafa et al. (2009) access to further training ranks among the priorities of middle cadres of the Malawian health workforce, making clear that the recently graduated nurses share the strong motivation to seek professional development with other nurses and health professionals in Malawi. However, as the above discussion has highlighted, their biographical (hi)stories as well as their family and peer group environments shape particularly strong self- and social expectations towards future educational and professional career attainment, which reflect in their concrete life plans and professional priorities. The professional self-identity of the students is to be understood as an academic one in the first place and this establishes linkages between the students' professional identity and their aspirations towards migration-to-study projects, tackled in the next chapter.

### *The Yearning for Migration-to-Study*

The central role of migration-to-study in the students' professional projects explains partly in view of the trapped situation they face in Malawi at their current point in career. Firstly, Master programmes in Malawi are full-time courses with high student fees, which blocks the option to work and study, making admissions selective to those with access to savings or loans.

Secondly, the students face a huge competition for the increasing, yet still very small number of Master programmes open to nurses in Malawi, covering in 2012 less then 35 places altogether: MSc Public Health (since 2003), MSc Midwifery (since 2009), MSc Reproductive Health (since 2010) and MSc Child Health Nursing (since 2010, in partnership with the University of Cape Town). This competition extends beyond their cohort and professional group: in the Master of Public Health, nurses compete with all other BSc graduates from the health sector, in particular with physicians. All other Master courses require a certificate in Midwifery, to be obtained in a 1-year certificate course necessary to gain the title of a Registered Nurse-Midwife. The certificate is not yet included in the students' Bachelor programme of General Nursing and the students were hardly able to estimate when they would get a chance to enter the course due to a limited number of places and a course cancellation in the previous years.[6] On behalf of continued education programmes in the public health service, a growing number of already experienced nurses have furthermore been trained at Bachelor level in a "post-basic" course at UNIMA. They present a further competitor of BSc Nurses regarding the admission to the local health-related Master Programmes, as the application processes consider examination performance, years in service and professional qualifications.

Though opportunities to do Master studies in Malawi are thus rare and the access to them socioeconomically selective, almost all participating students consider academic titles beyond the Bachelor level as an essential element of their profession projects, adding further to the fierce competition. In this situation, the low probability of admission to a Master programme in Malawi translates at the individual level into insecurity about the realization of the educational and professional project, and a resulting vulnerability of the overall life plan. Many students describe their migration projects within this context as a necessity (rather than a mere opportunity) to reduce this vulnerability and satisfy their self-expectations to become highly skilled professionals.

Seeking migration for professional development, they repeat a common scheme of nurse migration for further studies, which has been identified as one of the main reasons for migration among UK's overseas nurses from different origins (Alonso-Garbayo and Maben 2009; Buchan et al. 2006; Grigulis 2010). Concrete inducements for migration concern the wish to specialize in professional areas not offered in Malawi (e.g. MSc in Community Nursing or Psychiatric Nursing), and the expectation to find study and work environments that would enhance new professional inspiration and opportunities to improve one's practical qualification. Several stu-

---

[6] They might find themselves in an unfortunate position, as the still waiting previous cohort could be admitted first, while the cohort following them will advance directly into the position of a Registered Nurse-Midwife, following a new curriculum.

dents even express that they would prefer further training abroad and abstain from applying for local Master's, because they wished to find a new professional environment, better styles of teaching and a supervision that would give more recognition to their own learning goals.

The majority however is worrying first and foremost to find access to any Master programme because they do not expect to score high enough to compete successfully for one of the few study places. Not being among the best graduates of the year, they fear up to 10 years waiting time before admission to a Malawian Master programme, bringing the professional progress into conflict with other life projects. Contrariwise, the expected conditions of further education in the UK include the broad availability of study programmes and colleges, lower school fees and easier access to scholarships as well as the possibility to combine work and study. Against this background, even students with negative attitudes and expectations towards the personal experiences and challenges of migration consider a migration-to-study project.

Beyond the original biographic value of education, the students hold high expectations in the career effects of a Master's title, which explain from the perception that it would further validate and *institutionalize* their status as a highly skilled health professional. According to Bourdieu (1986), *not-institutionalized* cultural capital is constantly required to prove itself and therefore vulnerable to dequalification, while academically sanctioned cultural capital is, instituted by "*collective magic*" (Bourdieu 1986: 51), formally independent from the person of its bearer and legally connected with different entitlements to access higher positions and remuneration on the labour and social market. In the nursing students' career context however, the cultural capital of their Bachelor's degree proves little valuable and requires a socially higher valued and less contested international title-upgrade to be translated into attractive job positions and social and economic well-being. As outlined by one student, the aspired social position and professional status prove even more relevant to the idea about the value of institutionalized education than the expected financial gains:

“Researcher: So further study leads to money?

Participant 26F: I also think, but less important, it leads to “self fertilization”[?]. You feel like at least I've reached something to be satisfied.

Participant 29F: And you are also educated. For example after doing Master's, when you come back here to Malawi, you become a boss; you have your work done by others. [some laugh and giggle]

Participant 30F: I think, as she said, it sounds different, if you own a Dr. [Veronica], you get very much honoured by that! But if you are called Professor Veronica [gesture expressing: you reach the peak]!” [name changed] (WS 4: 9)

These thoughts about the benefits from education abroad mirror closely the spectrum of aspects in Marshall's definition of the drivers of professional status:

“(1) ‘market situation’ entailing an individual’s ‘economic position’, shaped by ‘source and size of income, degree of job-security and opportunity for upward occupational mobility’; (2) ‘work situation’, meaning the ‘set of social relationships in which the individual is involved at work by virtue of his or her position in the division of labour’ and (iii) status situation denoting the individuals’ position ‘in the hierarchy of prestige in the society at large’” (Marshall 1998 quoted in Aboderin 2007: 2240).

Capitalising on migration, the strategy to develop one's professional and social status with advanced education expands into the transnational field: working and studying abroad is expected to ameliorate the professional status, promising upon return occupational conditions associated with economic and social capital benefits and securities. Where the educational system abroad is prestigious among Malawians, the Master's title from abroad is expected to generate a distinctive status, as is the case for Master's from the UK, the colonial source country of the Malawian educational system (Grigulis 2010).

Interestingly, the expectation of status improvement contrasts sharply with the experienced professional development opportunities of overseas nurses in the UK. Former studies document instead experiences of professional and social status loss of African overseas nurses, up to the point of an "*embodiment of discrimination*" (Larsen 2007: 1). This unbars an immense gap between migration intentions driven by the imperative of status generation, and migration experiences of status deprivation in the destination country context. Findings of Grigulis (2010) point in particular to the difficulty to pursue studies while covering the daily needs and sending money home, which frequently leads to failure or endless prolongations of nurses' migration-to-study projects. Malawian research findings furthermore question the students' perception that a Master's degree would play a decisive role for career promotion in Malawi's health system (Tambulasi and Chasukwa 2011; MSH 2009; RoM et al. 2007). To my knowledge there are no statistics on the academic status of personnel in Malawi's higher health administration and in ministerial positions. The afore mentioned studies find that inefficient personal management structures for higher cadres, including the ministerial level, hamper the career development of Master's degree holders.

The not-anticipated risks of status loss abroad on the one hand, low status potential of the academic degree on the other hand bear a fundamental threat of failure to the students' professional migration-to-study biographic projects. At the same time, the huge gap between the anticipated benefits of migration and academic titles, and the lived situation of migrating nurses, point to the illusionary character of the biographic narration on migration, loaded with a socially transferred glorifying imagination of migration. One concrete aspect of this is the nurses' idealistic narrative about the UK as place to practice "*the ideal nursing*"[7] learned at university. They explain their vision of Britain as the ideal place for nursing contrasting with resource-scarce working settings in Malawi, where

---

[7] Recurrent statement in workshop questionnaires (Statements on "*What do you think about migration?*") and students' written documentation of small group discussions (Written statements: "*Motivations to migrate*")

the taught procedures were often inapplicable and improvisation and quality of care losses marked the daily experience.

A deeper meaning of the idea is however tangible when considering the (post)colonial link of (nursing) education in Malawi, which has always followed a British education system and curriculum for the Bachelor of Nursing (Grigulis 2010). The association between British nursing and *the ideal nursing* presented at university transfers the colonial idea about the superiority of British knowledge and practice in nursing to Malawian students, who thus associate opportunities to study and work in the UK with the privilege of gaining a status superior to local nurses. The inherent devaluation of local nursing knowledge repeats patterns of the colonial occupation of knowledge: the power relations inherent in colonialism transported a notion of superiority and truth, with which imperial nursing was imposed on the colonized and their local knowledge (Hallam 2000). The students' high expectations to "*get the sense of appreciation*"[8] when working abroad, contrasting sharply with the actual experiences of many African overseas nurses in the UK, reflect the standing of imperial nurses, white middle-class women who introduced nursing as a prestige profession for their compeers and a selection of black middle-class women (Hallam 2000; see p. 25). Larsen et al. find similar premigratory imaginations among South African overseas nurses, underlining the existence of a widely spread myth of British nursing:

"'Oh, this is where we learn everything from.' And so I expected to learn a lot and be able to take back something to South Africa. (Female, 50 years old, South African, white, D grade)";

"I was just expecting everything, as I say, a higher standard because we're told 'Oh, where you are going.' [...] and you just say 'Oh, I do like England. I am going somewhere.' (Female, 54 years old, South African, black, D grade)" (Larsen et al. 2005: 360).

---

[8] This expression occurred repeatedly in the workshops regarding nurses' general motivation to go abroad, as well as in their personal reasoning and expectations (Written statements).

Colonial images of British nursing join here a *myth of migration* (Dannecker 2009, see below) built over generations of nurse migration of Malawi. Several interviewees [9] referred in their descriptions about common migration intentions among Malawian nurses to overwhelmingly positive experiences of other nurses abroad, contradicting the picture emerging from the studies referenced above. The frequent citation of positive experiences stresses in this context the necessity to approach the illusionary character of migration intentions with regard to the long-lasting tradition of nurse migration from Malawi and the abundance of positive social narrations of migration surging from it. Stories of former generations of nurses abroad may lead to a continuous reproduction of mythic connotations between professional progress and social prestige, blurring the migrants' concrete experiences. This may be explained in view of the risk of deviant stories of failure to destroy the migrants' symbolic capital, making overseas nurses unfree to talk about their problems abroad and instead inclined to report only the expected personal success stories of migration.

The biased images evoked back home in turn contribute to the construction of a *myth of migration*, as has also been found by Dannecker (2003) in the context of women's labour migration from Bangladesh to Malaysia.

„Regardless of the experiences and the social and economic realities the migrants are confronted with abroad, a social behaviour, namely a specific way to narrate the migration experiences, accompanies migration and return, leading to the reproduction of the myth of migration.“ (Dannecker 2009: 14)

This situation is likely to apply in the context of Malawian overseas nurses, who need to bridge a similarly huge gap between social expectations and actual opportunities abroad as is the case for Bangladeshi migrants: Grigulis (2010) has highlighted that many find themselves confronted with overwhelming family expectations of support to which they try to conform in order to avoid disappointment and secure their position in the family. Disregard-

---

[9] Particularly Interview P5M; also Interviews P2F and P36F

ing the challenges they faced abroad, they maintained euphemistic images about the wealth, working and living conditions of migrant nurses towards those seeking migration, as uncovering the myth was expected to be dismissed as envy to see others equally well-off:

"[...] they will say I discouraged them and I am doing better, built houses, and I have got a car, and they haven't had a chance to come here because I told them it's a horrible place. How come I am able to stand this horrible place?" (Lindiwe quoted in Grigulis 2010: 187)

The imperial legacy of nursing and the dynamics upholding a *myth of nurse migration* have established a historical association between the prestigious status of nursing in the *West* and the common idea that migration increases nurses' professional capacity, increasing young nurses social status expectations connected with migration. Building on this social imagination, the individual nurses' prospects of exposure to a modernized nursing system overseas *and* an upgrade of personal educational capacities, represent exclusive privileges. Jointly they are expected to add up to build a valuable *symbolic profit of distinction* in the Malawian society (see p. 77), attributing the opportunity of migration-to-study an outstanding biographic value to further one's occupational and social future perspectives.

Less determining of the nurses' biographic orientation, yet still of interest in this context, is a second linkage between migration and nursing, which does not relate to nursing students' occupational ambitions but to the professional ethics of nursing:

"On nursing as a profession in terms of migration it's important, because nurses, we are not limited. Everywhere you can care for people as long as it is a person: We can care. So whether you are abroad or stay in the country, but if you are a nurse, you can care." (WS 1, P4F: 1)

Regarding the general life plan ambiguity surging from the ethical dilemma between making one's contribution in Malawi and taking the chances abroad (see p. 65-66), several women nurses turned the professional universal ethos of nursing into a moral legitimation for migration using this argument: in Workshop 4, when exposed to text passages questioning the ethics of nurse migration from a moral and humanitarian point of view, students countered that from their understanding the nature of nursing was to care for sick humans, regardless of their country or context (see p. 135). While sharing ethical concerns towards migration on a personal and social level, they adopted a positive, religiously tinted moral attitude towards the migration of nurses in general, in counter-balance to the public expectation that Malawian nurses should serve Malawians.

### Gender and Professional Identity

While the attractiveness of migration revealed as a cross-gender phenomenon among the students, the 'gender of nursing' and the students' gendered professional identities shaped the role of migration in their respective professional life projects tangibly. A historical perspective on nursing as a profession is helpful to contextualize the students' gendered approaches to nursing and migration. Studies on the *feminization of nursing* have evidenced how the professional status of nursing among health professions as well as today's public images about nursing stand in continuity with the nursing reforms introduced by Florence Nightingale in the late 19th's and the beginning 20th's century, reproducing images of femininity and female work of that time (e.g. Mackintosh 1997; Evans 2004). On the level of the individual nurse, good feelings when caring for others and an emotional and altruistic aspect of giving appeal to a self-perception in the classical terms of femininity (Hallam 2000; Schultheiss 2010). Nursing furthermore continues to carry a religious connotation with nurses being portrayed as female servants of God:

> "In the spirit of Florence Nightingale's life and writings, choosing to be a nurse began to be portrayed as a calling or a response to a higher being […]" (Brodie 1994 quoted in Magnussen 1998: 175).

As discussed earlier (see p. 25), the female missionaries introducing nursing in Malawi embodied these concepts of nursing, which are still persistent in today's public image of Malawian nurses. This becomes tangible e.g. in the illustration of a nurse as a female angle in a campaign in 2010 by the Malawian nurses' syndicate NONM titled "Soon there will be no angels on earth" (Picture 1). Several female students appealed to the link of professional and religious self-identity, describing professional satisfaction in pursuing a caring mission, which God had called them personally into, and a gratification and emotional commitment when curing patients and nursing "*from the heart*" (Interview P25F: 17).

*Picture 1. NONM Billboard Advertisement in 2010*

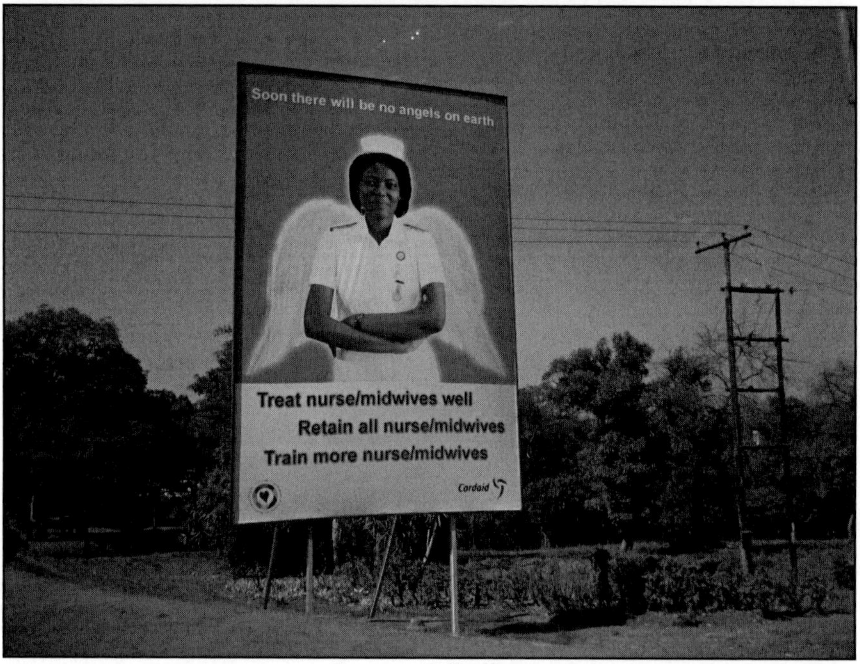
Soon there will be no angels on earth
Treat nurse/midwives well
Retain all nurse/midwives
Train more nurse/midwives
Cordaid

Source: Dibelius

Growing into nursing was furthermore connected with an affirmation of the personal gender-identity of becoming a *real lady*: "*Though I did not choose it, like everybody, I now like it, because it's like I become a real lady.* " (WS 1, P3F: 6) Female nursing students reported that, throughout the years of studies, they had developed a fundamental identification with their role as caregivers. This identification went beyond the level of aspirations towards status and career but developed from the perception that nursing was their professional calling (e.g. Interview P25F and P2F). As already treated earlier (see p. 80-81), several female interviewees reported on a difficult time of adaptation, marked by fears before patients and hospitals, lack of knowledge about the nursing profession and demanding learning-expectations at KCN, Interview P2F and P25F). Despite these initial challenges to adapt and the described frustrations about working- and career conditions, they expressed by the end of their studies a strong identification with their professional life as nurses, reflecting in many statements that they would make the choice for nursing again (e.g. WS 1). This circumstance suggests that their professional compromise, nursing, gained sustainable viability due to factors beyond the occupational prospects and points to the impact of socially defined anchors of identification, interweaving professional, religious and gendered identity.

Applying Bourdieu's concept about the convertibility of capital in social fields of power (1986) to the situation of female graduates in nursing in Malawi, several social advantages of women nurses reveal. Compared to their male colleagues and other women in the country, they secure a relatively high degree of symbolic capital in their profession: the exceptionality of their cultural capital, institutionalized by their academic title, elevates them noticeably from the average Malawian woman, holding a *scarcity value* which secures additional material and symbolic profits to those possessing distinctively large cultural capital (Bourdieu 1986: 49; see p. 77). At the same time and in contrast to male nurses, they conform to the socially defined gender of the profession, which earns them the *symbolic capital of normality, "the privilege of comme il faut, conforming to the norm, and therefore enjoying a symbolic profit of normality"* (ibid. 1989: 69). Last but not least, they profit from the symbolic capital attached to nursing as a *Western* medical profession of privileged and skilled women, materializing in the social admiration for women nurses' white nursing uniform (Grigulis 2010). In view of these aspects, women nurses accordingly secure a relatively high status security, which might explain why several female interviewees (though not those with

PHD aspirations) were more optimistic than their male colleagues to find alternatives of professional development, if they could not find access to a master programme, e.g. combining nursing and business activities or working in NGOs.

Due to the highly gendered social connotation of nursing as a female profession, different conditions of professional identification emerge in the case of male nursing students: as already mentioned, almost all male participants stated that they had entered nursing with the aim to get accepted to the physicians' programme, following a public rumour that the careers could easily be switched (see p. 81). When accepting to study nursing, they neither evaluated the profession as a long-term career option nor a prophecy, approaching the nursing programme instead as a temporary, strategic deviation towards their original professional choice. As they became aware of the career-switching rumour being false, the deflection of their professional project happened gradually and remained frustrating:

> "I think, I would really take another choice, because, as I earlier said, the attitude that the public and those in authority hold against us, male nurses, isn't all that impressive. So, given other opportunities I would really distance from that profession so that maybe I become what I want and so maybe I'll run away from this feeling of disefficiency in me. [...] Not satisfied really and not feeling full, like complete. Yes! [...]" (WS1, P6M: 5-6)

Male students' descriptions of discrimination as nurses suggest that conflicts of the gendered professional identity and frustrations at different levels accumulated throughout the years of study: many male workshop participants pointed to severe problems to be respected as male nurses in a profession socially classified as female, and as caregivers in the Malawian context where women are attributed the social role to care. Congruent findings by Grigulis (2010) may highlight the latter:

> "[...] in Malawian culture the caring role is done by the woman, so it is hard to accept a man as the carer. Even if their wife is sick the husband will not care for the wife, he will get female friends and relatives to look after her." (Female nurse in Grigulis 2010: 161)

Concretely mentioned manifestations of disregard or discrimination concern that male nurses were rejected by patients, faced public fleer for being a nurse and for wearing the nursing uniform, as well as disadvantages in career promotion (WS 1-3, Grigulis 2010). As the different incidences suggest, patients', colleagues and general social images of masculinity enter into conflict with the social image of nurses, which leads to reluctance to value male nurses' work and respect their male gender identity: Grigulis (2010) finds that male nurses were regarded as inferior to other male health workers and even openly treated as gay in a country where homosexuality is still legally punished. In view of these circumstances, the severe challenge of male nurses to identify with their professional role without loosing social status is self-evident. In reaction to the social stigma and as a consequence of male nurses' own concepts of gender, a large group of male research participants thus dissociated from the nursing profession, devaluating its caring character with gendered attributions:

> "Then I would choose another masculine course because for me nursing is more superficial, because it doesn't help me to think more deeper into my (subject?), so that I should choose a more masculine process so that I should at least look to myself as that I am a man again. (laughs, others join). That would be pleasant for me (?). Probably I would choose to go to College of Medicine, to do a bachelors degree in medicine, a bachelors degree in surgery for 5 years at least, so that is the way I would be satisfied." (WS 1, P5M: 5-6)

Such statements also reveal the persistence of ideas of male intellectual superiority and the inferiority of care work among highly educated Malawian men. Male students tended to maintain their gender-typical professional preferences (physician, surgeon, technician) over the time at KCN. E.g. one male interviewee stated that he aimed to practice two years in a welcoming hospital he already knew, before sidestepping the nursing profession via an educational upgrade into public health. At the time of graduation, being a nurse was still only acceptable as a temporary stage of career to far most male students, hoping to open doors to other, male-connoted occupations in health soon. They tended to express a more urgent need to find chances of further study to develop into male-type areas of the health sector such as science, management and politics. The overall impression gathered from research workshops and interviews was that most males aimed to proceed as fast as possible into health management professions via a Master's degree in Public Health. Among the three male interviewees two expressed little commitment to finish their years of duty if opportunities to leave Malawi for Master studies would show. Only one male participant described a deviant professional story, revealing an intrinsic motivation for and attachment to nursing, despite his plan to continue with reproductive health research and reach for a position in the Ministry of Health (Interview P15M). Three eventual reasons for his identification as a nurse may be relevant in his case: firstly, a personal and religious vocation towards helping needy people; secondly his extraordinary success in nursing, being receiver of several awards and an internship scholarship; and thirdly his positive experiences of professional development in nursing during his internship in Finland, in particular the assistance and supervision to pursue personal learning goals he enjoyed there.[10] His case suggests that a personal, in his context religious affiliation to the nursing mission and social appreciation for his professional performance as a nurse, characteristics found for most women nurses, can be helpful in generating professional commitment and *ownership* among male nurses as well.

Most male nurses however find themselves trapped professionally, which frames their migration-to-study projects differently from those of women nurses: in male nurses' biographic projects, migration becomes an essential means of status rehabilitation, sought not only to institutionalize their cultural capital of education, but also to regain the lost *symbolic profit of normality* with a professional activity in a male-connoted area of the health sector. On the contrary, in women nurses' projections migration is thought to improve the professional status and deepen the professional expertise as a nurse. In line with this, most of the female interviewees

---

[10] He reported to have been very inspired by the different learning environment focusing on personal priorities.

see their professional future after a return to Malawi in work fields related to nursing: among the interviewees, two women considered a return to the bedside in the area of psychiatric nursing and one woman sought to work with patients and in higher functions. The remaining hoped to find themselves in managerial positions, dealing with health-prevention, advocacy work, teaching or politics. Also those, however, who did not envisage a return to the bedside hoped to make valuable contributions via specialized nursing skills, new approaches to care, health care investments and nursing policy advocacy. In this context, they seek migration and further studies as a means of professional empowerment, creating entitlements to make a change in the profession and opening more satisfying professional prospects in Malawi:

"Participant 2F: I could say, what is more important to me is changing the profession [as compared to go forward in nursing studies]. But then, there are a lot of constraints here in Malawi, like challenges. Because you can have the desire to change the profession in our hospital setting, but then, maybe because of lack of resources, or maybe because of some other political factors, it's somehow difficult.

Researcher: Mhm. So you are not very optimistic about it? (Participant: Yes.) Would you say it's more on the dream-side then on the reality-side? (Participant: Yes, laughing) So do you think getting a Master's will give you better chances to pursue this dream? Or do you think you would rather be going into other areas to find what you are looking for in terms of professional development?

Participant 2F: If I find a chance, to pursue in this profession: I think I can be able to achieve that.

Researcher: But would you say it's your priority or do you think: I don't have to work in nursing.

Participant 2F: No, it's my priority! [...] I believe that when I go abroad I am going to gain some new knowledge, like in the nursing profession. Of which I believe that if I can come back with that knowledge and utilize it here in Malawi: I think then there can be some changes in the nursing profession. Yeah, that's what I believe." (Interview P2F: 10-11)

As the discussion of gendered preconditions of professional identity and biographic outlook has pointed out, male and female migration projects are integrated into different concepts of the professional future. It has become obvious that the intertwining of gender and religious identity with the professional attributes of nursing facilitate respectively challenge the generation of a biographic outlook in nursing. Though male and female students share fundamental scripts of professional identity as academics, their different positions towards a career as nurses is likely to have an impact on their retention in nursing and the potential of *brain gain* for nursing care in Malawi.

Notwithstanding this, the gendered contexts of Malawian nurses' migration projects have apparently not let to quantitative imbalances: while a survey by the Royal College of Nursing in the UK (quoted in Buchan and Dovlo 2004) points to a slightly higher share of men among overseas nurses as compared to the domestic gender balance in nursing, data reviewed by Tambulasi and Chasukwa (2011) does not support the existence of a gender disproportion for the case of nurse migration from Malawi.

It also should be mentioned that the evidently negative portent of overseas nurses' migration-to-study projects might also unsettle the identification of women nurses with their profession at a later stage in their professional biography. This is to be considered in particular as female gender has been found to fuel professional discrimination and reinforce a vicious circle of embodiment of discrimination abroad (Larsen 2007; Smith and Mackintosh 2007).

## The Partnership & Parenthood Project

The students' overall situation and future ideas on partnership/marriage and parenthood can be summarized as follows: None of the students talked to was married or had children. While the majority stated having a boy-/girlfriend or fiancé(e), 9 out of 39 participants stated to be single.[11] Among the interviewees, 4 persons (1 man/ 3 women) did not have a partner, while 6 persons (2 men/ 4 women) were in relationships with other university graduates[12], often nurses as well. Most interviewees were planning to postpone marriage and the foundation of a family until they would have finished their Master's degree. Others sought to marry within the next 2-3 years and have one child before going for further education, considering having more children later eventually. Among the single interviewees 2 stated they aimed to have a partnership after finishing their Master's degree, while 1 envisaged to stay single and 1 felt undecided in this question. Approaching the role of migration in students' partnership and parenthood life projects, it is of importance to clarify the gendered social context within which they develop their related biographic perspectives. The position of partnership and parenthood in the life plan reflects social conditions, which shape individual concepts of partnership and migration differently. Social expectations towards marriage and having children intertwine with related societal gender norms in shaping the students' visions of marriage and parenthood.

Despite the decreasing share of married women in Malawi[13], marriage is still an important social norm among Malawians and the expectation to get married is common in Malawi's educated classes as well: a tracer study of Kadzamira (2003) points out that the average number of singles among university graduates is similar to those of the overall population. Though advanced levels of education delay the age at first marriage usually until three years after graduation (ibid.), in 2004 tertiary educated women married with 22.6 years on average (Palamuleni 2011) and accordingly at the age of the study participants. Though none of the students was

---

[11] The number of singles among the workshop participants might be overestimated as some students with a boy- or girlfriend stated to be single because there partnership had not been formalized so far.

[12] One male participant did not specify whether his girlfriend was a graduate.

[13] In 2010 58% (2004: 67%) of all Malawian women between 15 and 49 were married, 19,7% (2004: 17%) had never been married, compared to 39,4% (2010) of men in the same age group (Mahowe 2005; NSO/ICF Macro 2011).

married as the point of the study, marriage revealed as a core element of most individual life plans. The study participants' ideas of parenthood reflect the general trends among highly educated Malawians to have fewer children: Palamuleni (ibid.) reports a significantly reducing effect of education on fertility rates, which had already been stated in 2003 by Kadzamira, finding that university graduates had 1.3 children on average seven years after their graduation.

A strongly gendered picture emerges, when looking into the consequences of social expectations on marriage and parenthood. The statement of a male students highlights that conformity to the social expectation of marriage is required to escape scorn and gain the social recognition attributed to a married man:

"Participant P5M: Since here in Africa marriage is one of the societal components which is being, which is valued most, to stay maybe up to 30 without getting married, people, maybe parents, ladies start to question the guys impotence (laughing), that sort of thing. So you need to prove that you are a man, to get married as early as possible. So when I finish school, in three years time, I need to get married.

Researcher: So you want to conform to this expectation?

Participant P5M: Ya ya, I have to. Because when you are a married man, in African societies you are MUCH respected. When you have a child, you are much respected. Instead if you are just staying alone, they will not respect you. So you need to conform to those societal expectations." (Interview P5M: 6)

In the Malawian context of a patriarchal society, married men are attributed social privilege as a symbolic capital, and gain individual authority: another male student highlighted that the institution of marriage is regarded as a prerequisite for men to decide and plan independently of the family of origin (Interview P5M). With respect to individual migration decisions, conformity to the principal of marriage is thus likely to contribute in the case of male nurses to the flexibility to take decisions for migration and return, as far as the societal influences are concerned.

Malawian women find themselves in a more ambivalent situation as gender roles in marriage establish new patterns of dependence and subordination that may affect their scope of action, e.g. regarding migration decision-making (Grigulis, Prost and Osrin 2009). The strongly restricted life planning entitlements of women until marriage suggest that being unmarried is associated with a high influence of the family of origin (see p. 61). Upon marriage, the family's influence tends to be transferred to the husband, rather than to the woman herself, as suggested by the MDHS 2010 general findings on decision-making patterns in Malawian marriages. High influence on household decisions is found mainly among divorced, separated or widowed women, when correlating with advanced age and number of children, low education, own cash earnings and an urban background (Mahowe 2005).

While education and single status do not improve the lamentable decision-making status the young nurses share with women in their age group in general, looking beyond the current age, the statistics document a high entitlement to participate in household decisions among married, tertiary educated women with children who have own income (NSO/ICF Macro 2011). This points to fortunate conditions of empowerment for female university graduates - if they accept marriage and parenthood as part of their future life plan. At the same time, the expectation of the public life course to get married and have children constitutes an unavoidable challenge to female students' migration-to-study plans:

> “ I want to have at least one [child within the next years]. Because...- I understand that there are some complications if I have a child and I (migrate from here?). But there are several complications that happen here in Malawi, or in a woman. So I don't want to have those complications, I just have to have just one, so I should know that: I think I'm fertile (laughs).” (Interview P32F: 14)

This statement hints at a negative general opinion on childlessness, but also the status of single woman, which both are looked upon as considerable personal deficiencies (Mahowe 2005), connected with negative image consequences.[14] This became tangi-

---

[14] The design of the MDHS 2010 is meaningful in this regard as it does not attribute any attention to the decision-making situation of unmarried women.

ble for example when a leader of a nursing organization, herself a highly educated nurse with international experience, was deeply shocked by the fact that the nursing students talked to had not yet been married and tended to postpone marriage intentions to the time after their master studies.

### *Couples' Migration Projects*

Approaching from here the life projects of partnership and migration among female students with a boy friend and a marriage plan, an ambiguous picture emerges. On the one hand, none of them mentioned fears to loose sight of the professional plans when married. Even when having a child while still studying was regarded as a challenge, they expected to cope with it, counting on mutual solidarity within the couple (e.g. P2F, 210F): as the interviews revealed, the common idea on how to cope with the challenge that both partners aimed to advance their educational status while having responsibilities for a family, was either that one partner should work and take care of the family while the other one could go for further studies and vice verse, or that the male partner should leave in order to prepare the following of his wife or family.

Women nurses were confident that role-switching in the couple (working, studying, and taking care of children) would be supported by their partners and that those were compliant to the common life plan, e.g. in making mutual investments into the other's education or having common business investments. Only one woman expected the situation to be challenging, which made her undecided on when to marry, when to go abroad and when to do master's.

At the same time several interviewees expressed ambitious self-expectations to pursue their professional objectives if they were not able to count on the husband's equal involvement (e.g. Interview P32F, P10F), as well as to defend their ideas about family life assertively vis-à-vis their partners. Most of the interviewed women who were in a partnership had chosen first working places located relatively far from their partners', which may be seen as an indicator for their current decision-making focus on professional opportunities, rather than the needs of the partnership. As female interviewees' partners are without exception university students or degree holders who favour migration, the common wish to study abroad translates into several couple migration projects. Though most students did not specify whether they would go one after the other, or whether the first to leave would facilitate the partner' migration later, the partnership becomes in these cases a pro-migratory factor supporting the young women's plans to further their education abroad.

A closer look at the couples' migration projects however questions women's equal preconditions to pursue their personal agenda of migration, suggesting a tendency among women nurses to postpone own projects of further education and migration and subordinate them to those of their partners: one female student was informed by her partner that he was arranging to go abroad, but would only tell her more when everything would be fixed. While she perceived this situation as positive because she assumed it to enlarge her opportunities to migrate, she was not given the opportunity to participate in decision-making. In two cases, where both partners were nursing graduates at the same point in career, they had agreed that the male partner should try to migrate first for his girl friend or wife to follow him when he had managed to settle. These situations remind of the "*following spouse*" scheme of women nurses, found by Muula, Nyasulu and Msiska (2004b: 76) regarding the process of rural-urban migration: the authors observe that women nurses in Malawi tend to follow their husbands, i.e. change (and thereby subordinate) their professional and living environment to their husbands' ones, which adds to the problem of an uneven distribution of nurses in the country.

However, the women nurses' plans stand in another context than traditional patterns of migration, like migration to accompany a husband or reunify a family, in which women's movement is directed by a family agenda (UNFPA 2006). In the young nurses life projects, the partners' move abroad is linked to realizing the individual professional agenda and integrates well into the women's self-perception as ambitious, assertive and self-made. Nonetheless, the situations described above point to a gender gap in access to and *ownership* of migration-to-study projects among nurses living in a partnership or marriage.

Considering from here the women nurses' chances to pursue their migration intentions, it can be suggested that marital status, partners' migration projects and commitment to role-switching in the couple may constitute important factors at the point of decision-making for migration. Concrete choices of destination and the experiences and professional chances inherent to migration are likely to be reshaped not only by accessible options, but also according to male partners' priorities. At the same time, the couples' common migration projects can be conceived as a biographic strategy that allows pursuing individual professional goals while progressing in the common partnership and parenthood life project and foregoing the challenges of repeatedly mentioned fears of social isolation abroad.

### *Singles' Migration Projects*

While most singles interviewed envision to get married after finalizing their Master's degree respectively when financial independence would be obtained, two women dissociate themselves from the paradigm of marriage in stating that they could imagine or aim to stay single: one student (P31F) projects herself into a missionary life context where the status as single is likely to be socially justified. The other one (P36F) looks forward to a single's life abroad and prepares to confront social stigma in Malawi. A third woman considered staying single unless she finds the possibilities to realize a marriage matching her demands.

The latter two (P25F; P36F) were little optimistic with respect to their position as married women in Malawi and disclose a different approach towards partnership, parenthood and migration that will be explored in the following. They share the attitude that women in marriages were vulnerable to discrimination and abuse by Malawian men in terms of an unfair distribution of work, respect and financial means. In the case of P25F a central point of conflict emerged between what she considers the common culture in Malawi and her notion of equality between partners, involving mutual respect, financial independence and the sharing of household chores:

"[…] I want to have a microwave, my cooker and everything. Those I want to be in my kitchen, my sitting room, the way my room I want it to be; those things I have been dreaming of, those things I have been working for as in school, you see? Why? Because I have seen many people who suffer. Mainly it's on the side of ladies, where someone will come and then you are married and someone starts thinking: 'oh I am the one who did this!' But people even should be able to tell that ladies can be independent and you, if you meet a lady, don't think they are only workers, but they are people like you. You are there because you want people to be together and because of love, you see? [...] Because people think that women get married to be assisted. No! Even, the people, they use the word women as an acronym when they will say they are 'Workers of Men Employed Naturally', of which I say: 'why they say that?'" (Interview P25F: 8)

The priorities for a good marriage revealing here indirectly, intersect with the expectations of this nurse towards migration insofar as she presumes to meet more men abroad who would share these attitudes about women and partnership. She reports that her family used to have international visitors, coming to pray in her father's (Pentecostal) ministry and that male visitors expressed irritations about the unequal sharing of household labour in her family. She concludes from there that men in *Western* societies would hold more liberal and to her mind and lifestyle appropriate attitudes of gender equality, raising her attraction by a foreign life partner (Interview P25F). Her migration intention is formulated in an attitude of protest against subordination to what she perceives as a patriarchal local value system.

Furthermore, she approaches migration as a strategy to generate economic independence, which she regards as a precondition for an equal relation in a future marriage. Similar to her argument, several single nurses as well as nurses in a partnership pointed to the importance to generate personal savings to support children and partners (e.g. P27F, P5M). Gaining funds from migration to promote the personal status in the relationship was however mentioned by this nurse (P25F) only. Preferring migration as an option to realize her life project of partnership, she acknowledges that it would still somehow be possible to find the desired type of partner in Malawi as well.

To the contrary, one single nurse (P36F) did not consider a marriage with a Malawian man at all. While both expect to meet abroad men with different attitudes towards gender roles in marriages, P36F prefers to stay single there as well. In her case, the core conflict manifests between the social expectation to get married and take over the gender role of a wife on the one hand, and her wish to lead an independent life as a single woman on the other hand. She explains her negative attitudes towards marriage with respect to her negative biographic experience as child of an abusive father (she was raised by her mother who left the father and brought the children up under difficult economic circumstances. Her context makes a long-term migration project appear as option to forgo the stigma associated with being single in Malawi, maintaining the social peace back home while profiting from a social environment abroad where an independent lifestyle is expected to be normality:

> "I think the easiest way to live single will be abroad but here, because people will call you names. Yes, I may not mind but somehow it can have an effect on me, my parents, (people?) coming and saying: Hey, look at this. So being single in outside world there it would be very good, no problems, but, when it comes here down here – mhm – will be a problem I know, I am done and I am ready, I am prepare for it. […] Say, if I go outside there, stay single – for me it will be cool, because I will not have pressure from parents, friends, the society itself. It will be on me. So I would better run away from this, I would better go outside and stay there – come back – see them – go back." (Interview P36F: 15)

As the statement points out, young Malawian nurses may seek migration as a biographic strategy that goes beyond the prospect to find abroad more independence and acceptance for their personal way of life. Additionally, the move abroad is meant to create a distance that would protect one's own and the family's social capital and status.

Fleeing public stigma as a single woman has also been revealed as a pattern of migration to the UK among women from other regions (e.g. Izuhara and Shibata 2002 for Japan, UN-DESA 2005) suggesting that the idea of a good life for singles in the *west* forms part of a transnational body of images among women migrants. Next to the two cases discussed above, several students expressed ideas that women living in the UK or the USA had more entitlements in their destination societies (WS 5). It is possible that those images surge partly from what has been discussed in the literature as *social remittances*, i.e. changing ideas, behaviours and self-identities of gender equality surging from women's migration experiences (e.g. UNFPA 2006; Dannecker 2005; Larsen et al. 2005). Where social remittances are transferred back to the community of origin, they may challenge gender norms and introduce a body of images about migration and gender empowerment, as Levitt observed for Peruvian women migrating to the USA:

> "Due to their more active participation in public life in the United States, women modify their notions of what is right and appropriate, and they transmit these back to Miraflores. Non-migrant women use these social remittances to construct new versions of womanhood. While their ideas are somewhat romanticized, they still represent a significant shift in thinking about what it means to be a woman. […] They hear that many men clean, cook and shop in the U.S. These notions challenge their understandings of the meaning of marriage and motherhood and about what men and women's roles and responsibilities should be." (Levitt 1996: 15-16)

Whereas such imaginations may also be established via media and other channels of information, the strong culture of nurse migration from Malawi has most likely left its footprint here. In this regard, the cases of P25F and P36F illustrate that the fear before patriarchal limitations of women's rights in local marriages may have an implicit impact on migration intentions of women nurses who affiliate themselves to a global community of women claiming equal gender rights: their affinity to partners and societies assumed to share attitudes of gender equality and personal independence points to a *social space* of reference for their migration decision-making that transcends the local environment and extends into a global community of values. At the same time, their gender-related self-identities establish as counterpoints to what they regard as *local* culture, drawing instead on a *global* codex of entitlements of gender equality and self-determination (Bastia 2011).

Additionally to the prospect of self-empowerment discussed ahead, migration intentions of single nurses may also stand in the context of a struggle to find a life partner in Malawi: it is a common public assumption that female hospital nurses face particular difficulties to find attractive husbands due to their work in remote areas and in shift work (Grigulis 2010). The students referred e.g. to the absence of women over night and their low availability in the house due to long shifts and over-time work affecting their attractiveness in the eyes of potential husbands. One student group discussed this situation as the *nurses' syndrome* (WS 5), adding that nurses might seek to migrate to escape this dilemma and find a life partner there:

> "Because here in Malawi we have a certain thing which we call nurses syndrome. So people run away and go abroad to say here we have the syndrome, maybe I may not (find somebody?). We have that nurses' syndrome where nurses don't marry or men don't go after them, so they stay for years without getting no life partner, nothing. So they … (pointing over her shoulder with her hand)." (WS 5, P36F: 2)

This concern did not repeat during the interviews and is also not confirmed in statistics, which estimate the share of unmarried women among nurses to be similar to that of other health professionals in Malawi (CSR 2007). It might however become a factor for nurses' who face problems to find life partners in their later decision-making regarding migration and work place choices.

As the discussion has shown, the biographic functions attributed to migration in the context of future partnership and parenthood life projects depend on the current status of each student's relationship, as well as the individual evaluation of chances to achieve one's partnership priorities within the Malawian social and gender context: Single women with independent life scripts seek migration as a strategy to gain personal self-determination, emancipate from social expectations of marriage, and protect their social and economic status. Nurses in partnership, find migration to offer a comfortable perspective to attain professional goals while pursuing a common partnership and parenthood life project. Students seeking to migrate with their couple as well as single students with emancipatory gender identities tend to be more open towards extended stays as compared to students who envisage migrating without their partners or uphold close family contact as a central value (e.g. Interviews P31F; P32F).

In the light of the social context of gender relations in marriages in Malawi, the attitudes and biographic priorities of women nurses' partners are likely to influence the women's conditions to pursue individual biographic goals connected with migration. At the same time the high affinity to migrate among nurses' partners raises the chances to realize a migration project and points to the role of migration experience as part of a common habitus, thus supporting the argument that migration intentions have to be understood within the nurses' broader peer environment of young academics.

## Family Bonds

The extended family - i.e. the social structure within one household or a network of households, connected by kinship relations, common responsibilities and decision-making - presents as the core micro-social entity of social organisation and decision-making in the Malawian context (van Blerk and Ansell 2004; Kasente 2006). The embedding of the students' future life concepts within the context of their extended family, as well as within a core family understood as parents and siblings, reveals clearly in their biographic stories: The influence of the core as well as the extended family on fundamental biographic decisions and trends has been illustrated with regard to the process of career choice and encouragement towards education (see p. 75-76).

A strong and lasting intertwining between the students and their extended families became furthermore tangible on the level of the household's economy: Frequently students acknowledged that the investment of the (extended) family into their education should be paid back, e.g. supporting the schooling of siblings' children or supporting and caring for ageing or ill relatives. While parents were usually the central supporters of education, uncles and siblings had also contributed to school fees and living costs. In particular where parents only counted with modest means, the students had profited from the financial support of the broader family and assumed economic responsibilities extending over four generations, from grandparents over parents to siblings families. In the two cases where students' core families had faced periods of hardship (P31F and P36F), members of the extended family (grandmother, uncle) had even taken over the entire responsibility to care for the child, finance his or her education and provide moral and emotional guidance.

The experienced biographic importance of the extended family mirrors in the students' wider future life plans and the role attributed to family matters in their general life scripts and migration projects. Family authority and family values regarding the personal life plans, common attitudes towards the role of family in personal decision-making and the family-relatedness of the individual migration projects stick out as issues meriting further discussion, also with regard to specific dynamics of gender.

The family of origin is considered in the students' life plans as an important social bond and as an institution of authority. The wish to maintain a close relationship of mutual solidarity with family members is expressed by many students as an important aspect of a happy future life. Also, the contribution to family members' well-being, mostly financially but also psychologically and via nursing care, is an important consideration in most students' future plan. Students not carrying such responsibilities still severally highlight the emotional importance of the family community. While the core family is expected to be supportive of the individual migration project in most cases, some students were confronted with negative attitudes towards migration within their family.

### ***Between Solidarity and Independence***

All students aim at finding ways to maintain the well-being of and the harmony with family of origin while pursuing individual professional, personal and family plans. In line with this, solidarity with the family is approached in the students' life plans as an essential pillar of social reality that has to be in harmony with individual priorities to live happily.

"[...] I can say that I will do this or I will do that and some plans will also be limited to the family that I will have. Of course some of them will be discussed in the family circle, like when to go for school, who will start. Because my husband, my future husband, would also be educated." (Interview P32F: 12-13)

Thus, all students, women stronger than men, anticipate and consider the family's attitudes and needs when preparing future decisions. Parents are outnumbering other advisors by far among the female participants. According to the introductory questionnaire handed out in the workshops, almost all female students would ask their parents for advice when making a migration decision and several female interviewees highlight that important decisions would be discussed in the family circle (P10F, P27F). Male participants in turn seldom state to consult parents. The interviews revealed however that men might also discuss their migration prospects with the family in an attitude of whishing their support and understanding. One male student convinced his father on his migration plan, the remaining male interviewees seemed to consider their parents' attitude without consulting them directly, i.e. assuming certain family responsibilities when making their plans.

However, though the limitations of personal choices by a family context are acknowledged, aims to limit the influence of family members on the personal life course become obvious as well: several students' life plans are strongly informed by the striving for individual self-determination. This is tangible in the statement of a woman who clearly prioritizes her independence over the social status security her upper middle class family could have provided her with:

"I wouldn't even [work in my father's cabinet]. I don't even dream of working there. Because I don't think I can be comfortable to work in a place where my father is also working - I don't think I can be comfortable there. Yeah. At least I should be independent; I should be able to make my own decisions. Otherwise, if I tried to say I would be working with my father, then, if conflicts arise, they don't just end at the workplace but even at home. So I would just be working under pressure, just to please him. But deep down the heart I'm not satisfied." (Interview P2F: 30)

In all interviews tackling this topic, the students expressed assertiveness to pursue their personal goals in life and to negotiate the required freedoms of decision-making with family members, mainly parents, if they did not already hold liberal attitudes towards their children. In the question of final *ownership* of the personal future, the family's stake tends to be seen merely in *mutual advice and support*, while the *final decision-making power* is attributed to the individual person.

"But according to your plans, you also have plans to do things. You can't just be saying: Because you are expecting more from me, then I have to sacrifice myself to do what they want. No. You also have plans like I want to do this and this. The money, I have earned it, at the end I have to do it: A, B, C, D." (Interview P32F: 21)

While solidarity within the family is preserved as central value, it is here subordinated to personal *ownership* of decision-making and considered under the condition of compatibility to personal future aspirations. With respect to female graduates, such ideas about decision-making challenge the essential authority of family over young Malawian women's life, suggested by the previously cited MDHS statistics (see p. 61). They strengthen the suggestion that individual rather than collective future plans build the mainstay of the students' life script as has been argued in the initial subchapter of the data discussion. And this individualized mindset builds a fundament for the claim towards lifestyle decisions discussed in the following chapter.

Furthermore, it points to an intergenerational negotiation of decision-making entitlements, stressed by one interviewee (P27F) who states that she has to defend her professional and self-development plans in discussions with the broader family (including siblings families) who have high expectations of financial support from her, the most educated child.

On the basis of the highlighted role of family in students' scripts of life, the family orientation of their migration projects will be scrutinized in the following, showing variations according to the status of the students' family and their gender. It is suggested that the strong influence of family on life decisions leads students to attempt furthering their self-determination abroad. From there, the family-relatedness of students' migration projects is characterized and contrasted against related previous findings on nurse migration from Malawi.

A single female nurse emphasizes parental and social heteronomy of her life plan as a central reason to seek a life in a distant and distinct social context:[15]

> “Because there it’s their life, so you live your own life. While here, you live somebody's life, that's the thing here in Malawi: You live somebody's life, you live the life of your parents. Like you want to be there with them, yet your mind is somewhere else, very far, but you know I just have to do this for my parents, not for yourself. Our friends are lucky there, they do their things for themselves, not for their parents.” (Interview P36F: 14)

The striving not to loose *ownership* of her migration and future plan reflects in her statement that she would only confront her family with her migration plans when these were already settled (ibid.). In her view, the embedding into a local network of family obligation counters individual freedoms of decision-making, which are thus projected onto life in a distant *Western* country.

---

[15] The student did not state or implicitly suggest that the problem would be specific to a girls’ role in her family. Her statement is therefore discussed without reference to gender, though gender might be an aspect of concern in this context.

Several other students conceptualize migration similarly as a major biographic step towards an independent life insofar as it is expected to raise the individual self-reliability (maturity to live without family's help (P15M)), self-actualisation (individual freedom of lifestyle (P2F)) and financial independence (ownership of own funds (P32F; P5M)). These side-effects of migration on individual empowerment are documented recurrently in the literature on female migration and build upon the paradigm that spacial distance would weaken the constraints caused by social obligations and roles back home and thus strengthen the individual *ownership* of life (UN-DESA 2005; UNFPA 2006; Larsen et al. 2005).

The reasoning of P36F however inheres an ambiguity between the whish to liberate from family expectations towards the personal life course and the acknowledgement that family obligations persist also over distance. Her situation comprises furthermore that staying single is not necessarily connected with higher individual *ownership* of personal decisions for Malawian women in families who do not grant them authority of decision-making, confirming the previously cited findings of the MDHS (see p. 61). Her ambivalent statement suggests that family expectations may have a stronger effect on women nurses' later decision-making for migration and return than their emancipative self-concepts suggest.

"Researcher: […] you said you like Australia, Canada and USA. So if you found a good opportunity to study there, would it be attractive to you to stay longer or how do you see that?

Participant 36F: The lord provides good things, indeed, but some things drag us back. Ya, I can go there and say I want to stay longer. But one time you must come back home and do some other things. Your relatives call, your duties call, to see you, something like that. But I will not really say I go there then to stay for good. Yes, *I can*, but I still have to consider my relatives as well." (Interview P36F: 12) [Italian by the author]

In the economic realm, the migration project appears again in many life plans as a strategy to cope with overwhelming family expectations:

"[…] And the money you receive, it ends there. I can say it's not that much money for you to keep somewhere, because here in Malawi we are social beings, we live in an extended family that we appreciate. I have my niece, who needs my support, my mama, my father, my children, my in-laws from my brothers; you can live ten in a family, TEN people in ONE family. So that is difficult for the salary that I get here in Malawi to keep and then to go for school." (Interview P32F: 20)

Several students report that their parents' motivation to educate them was strongly related to the wish to secure the family's economic well-being, highlighting the impact of education on obligations towards the family. In those families, common among the interviewees, only some siblings have been successful in education, while others have children but little income, establishing their dependence on brother's respectively sister's financial support. The students' pronounced wishes to reserve funds for educational promotion, a good living standard of the future core family and own personal development aspirations appear illusionary in view of never-satisfied needs and expectations of the family.

Students facing such burdening family constellations with high expectations of financial support disclose the expectation that migration could enhance their economic independence. Anchored in the conviction that personal needs should be considered before those of the family, their reasoning follows the already mentioned paradigm of distance: the dilemma is relocated into a distant social space imagined not only as a fortuitous environment to generate savings but also as a space freed from family influence on and control over personal earnings:

"But when one is outside Malawi, then the money that you receive, it adds value, it's a bit, the money, when you change it to Malawian Kwacha, it's much. So if that person goes outside she maybe doing some peace work, like my husband goes out, goes for school, he may be able to do some peace works so that he may be saving some money. Because there it's only him, he is alone. You can be saving some money, you can be sending or he may even find that opportunity of helping me to further my education. Or if I work, I go there for school, I can also be sending some money here to Malawi, working part-time there, doing some part-time jobs. And then supporting this one or saving for him." (Ibid.: 20-21)

In turn, students from families with better socioeconomic conditions and high embodiment of education among siblings maintain that their relatives would not need or expect their financial assistance and that they could even expect further support from their parents (e.g. P10F, P2F). In this context, mutual family obligation turns into a capital rather than a burden in the first place: The network of kinship is likely to continue facilitating the access to economic, cultural and symbolic privileges (Bourdieu 1986), acting as a social capital to realize personal future aspirations and overcome financial barriers to migration easier. Under both socio-economic family conditions, the needful and the prosperous, family obligations act as a furthering factor of migration intentions.

***Gendered Obligations***

The literature on migration points to a broad spectrum of en-twinements of gender and family dynamics, shaping the individu-al's migration intentions and preconditions to migrate even where family solidarity is guiding migrants' perceptions and discourses:

„[...] although household members' orientations and activities may be guided by norms of solidarity […] they may equally be informed by hierarchies of power along gender and generational lines; thus the tension, dissention [sic.] and coalition building these hierarchies produce within the migration process.“ (Pessar 1999: 582)

„The family both defines and assigns the roles of women, which determine their relative motivation and incentive to migrate, and controls the distribution of resources and information that can support, discourage, or prevent migration.“ (Boyd and Grieco 2003: n.p.)

Mirroring the intertwining of gender with family obligations and responsibilities, the students' migration projects are affected by gendered expectations making a difference to female students' pre-conditions of and approaches towards migration. Firstly, a social association of being a woman with solidarity towards the family, secondly, the already discussed connotation of (nursing) care for the ill and elderly with female gender (see p. 93-95) are important in this regard.

As stressed by a female nurse from a family with low educational attainment, expectations towards women's care for family issues can have repercussions for the burden of family responsibility to be carried by female graduates:

> "[...] In Malawi we would believe that educating a girl child is like you have educated the whole country. Yes because women, we have passion to other people, helping other people (more) than men. So in families we believe educating the girl child is like you have educated the whole family: she can support, help the family in terms of needs." (Interview P27F: 1)

P27F explains that her siblings expect her to support their families substantially and that she expects fierce negotiations to win her family's endorsement for her personal projects e.g. when financial benefits from her migration would present. Her situation suggests that (specifically in poor families) educated girls might have to make more effort to gain authority over their earnings and life plans than men, disclosing an intersection of gender and class with respect to the value of family solidarity. In line with this, women overseas nurses from Malawi in the UK expressed that family members' often had overwhelming expectations that they could not satisfy unless distributing their resources at the expenses of their personal quality of life:

> "They end up relying on you and they expect money from you all the time so you are sort of the breadwinner for your family there. You have to pay your bills here and then you have to do it back home as well. It is difficult...that is why most people they have got their full time jobs but they do agency work as well or overtime bank. They end up doing extras every week to [...] send money home." (Statement of a female registered nurse in the UK quoted in Grigulis 2010: 194)

This situation reflects the general finding that the transnational extension of family obligations tends to shape especially women migrants' living conditions throughout their time abroad as women often "*struggled to retain the gains that migration and wage employment brought them*" (UN-DESA 2005: 63). Male migrants face a high burden of responsibility as well (e.g. Schraven, Eguavoen and Manske 2011 on male PHD students), however they tend to be able to retain more profits of migration for their personal life (UN-DESA 2005). Women migrants furthermore stick more closely to assigned responsibilities for the needy family than men tending to fall into the scheme of altruistic remittance senders: they attribute higher shares of their (on average lower) incomes to families far away remitting particularly for basic items such as health, education and nutrition, and supporting their families more reliably over long periods abroad (Moreno-Fontes 2008; Orozco, Lowell and Schneider 2006; UNFPA 2006). Some of this literature (e.g. UNFPA 2006) however tends to approach the topic under a biased perspective that reproduces rather than analyses gender roles: claiming/assuming that families and children left behind by mothers would suffer particularly from the distance, the idea is redone that women belong more closely to their families than men. In view of these patterns of expected solidarity and support, women among the nursing graduates who prioritize to generate savings are particularly likely to enter into conflict with their families.

The second challenge to women's migration projects concerns the already discussed gendered attributions of care. While these ease women's careers in the profession of nursing, they hold particular burdens for women nurses' migration projects as female relatives are expected to care for the ill or elderly in their family. This translates into mobility restrictions for women nurses and has been identified as a stick-factor in former generations of nurse migration from Malawi (Grigulis 2010). Male nurses with similarly struggling families were in turn not confronted with demands for their caring presence as their sisters were in charge of these tasks, maintaining the social gender order of care (ibid.). Studies on transnational caregiving have disclosed that obligations to care tie the individual's life course to the family life cycle as parents age or die or as migrants start to require family care themselves (Izuhara and Shibata 2002; Baldassar, Vellekoop Baldock and Wilding 2007). Thus, the family life cycle might determine the support for women nurses' migration in particular ways and shape their obligations of care while abroad, affecting their individual leeway of decision-making.

In accordance with these findings, women nurses who accept the assigned caring role in the family expect conflicts when pursuing individual priorities and migration projects in the future. Their internal dilemmas harden in cases where family members had convinced the woman to study nursing in order to assure care for ill parents (P32F), and where emotional attachment to an elderly person is guiding the future outlook (P31F). As can be concluded from these cases, the moral conflicts surging from caring responsibilities for family members tend to impact women nurses migration projects in duration, destination and character.

P32F highlights that in her future plan the expectations of a huge number of family members would have to be considered. While she accepts to be part of the system of family responsibility, this correlates with assumed difficulties to pursue own professional goals and generate savings to support the family she hopes to found in future. She questions her possibility to leave and expects to alternate with her partner (one furthering studies abroad, one assuming family responsibilities back home) if leaving at all (Interview P32F).

P31F has a widowed grandmother and is the only person who explicitly mentions the issue of care for the elderly as a factor acutely determining her migration outlook: she considers to postpone the migration project till the burden of responsibility would diminish, to restrict the choice of destination to closer (i.e. African) countries and to limit the time span abroad strictly to the time of studies. Other female students currently not concerned with caring obligations might be confronted with these in future, as the family life cycle proceeds and parents grow older. This would not necessarily mean a restriction to migrate as their social role as the best-educated child in the family might rather require them to care financially while female siblings take on the task of providing hands-on care.

Though all interviewees' life plans disclose an effort to build compromise between individual and family-related priorities that are seen as interlacing rather than opponent, the relation between family expectations and personal intentions bears potential for conflict in the case of women nurses. Interviewed men also point to high responsibilities to provide for family members, yet not describing conflicts but stating that they were successful in gaining the endorsement of their families for going abroad. This applies also in the case of a family with an elderly mother to be cared for, as the sister back home assumed the caring tasks (Interview P14F). As the family responsibilities highlighted by male nurses refer mostly to financial support, they expect to act in the common interest when seeking further education in order to establish in a professional position where they could assist their family considerably (Interviews P14M and P15M). In general, male interviewees tend to make their migration plans more independently, which suggests that their decision-making process for migration might be less tied to the family circle than that of their female colleagues.

### *Family Perspectives on Migration*

The overall picture emerging from this discussion on the family-relatedness of the students' migration plans distinguishes from the general finding of migration studies on the role of households in labour migration decisions. The *new economy of labour* theory on migration suggests that labour migration decisions should be approached as an economic survival strategy of entire households, assuming individual expectations towards migration to be situated within economic and status-related goals of the household or family (Arango 2000; Ramírez, Domíngues and Morais 2005). This has been supported by findings from Grigulis (2010) regarding former generations of overseas nurses from Malawi and applies, according to a key informant of the her study, also to the migration decisions of graduates from Kamuzu College of Nursing:

> "Most of them [KCN graduates] would be forced by their parents to go (to the UK). They want their children to be rich. There is a lot of pride if your son or daughter went to work in the UK because you are sure of the income aspect, they would be sending you money, you would be going to the UK to visit them, see London, who doesn't want to see London?" (Aubrey quoted in ibid.: 193)

Though the common perceptions of the students on nurses' reasons to migrate go into the same direction, none of the interviewees report on the existence of family pressure to leave in order to secure the family's well-being by means of migration. On the contrary, the described family attitudes on migration are largely ambiguous. Several students anticipate their parents to cast doubts upon their migration projects related to the fear to loose contact and support and to suffer emotionally from the distance (Quest.; WS 1). As various students mentioned, their mothers or fathers prefer their children to be successful within the country, establishing a patriotic reservation towards migration, claiming that *if you want to make it, make it here in Malawi.*[16] This variation of the students' idea that the best contribution is the one made in one's country (see p. 65-66) can be regarded as a reflection of an ambivalent social discourse on migration further discussed below (see p. 148-52). *'Making it'* abroad is discussed as the most viable and beneficial alternative; *'making it'* in Malawi (without leaving or upon return) however associated with particular social recognition.

It remains open whether the absence of direct family pressure to migrate goes back to the attitude that a Bachelor degree would be sufficient to acquire a job position securing the family well-being, which would be reasonable in view of the apparent advantages of university graduates on the Malawian labour market (Kadzamira 2003). Or whether parents' perspectives accentuate the dangers of migration, fearing unsuccessful migration projects in the young generation. The suggestion of some family members to take a sibling with them (Interview P5M and P2F) might then be regarded as a family strategy to avoid the risks of migration for the collective future, stabilizing family bonds abroad and increasing the collective profit from the assumed financial gains of migration. Family members alleged reluctance against migration should however not be overstated. Taking into account the enthusiastic social ideas of benefits from migration and the expectations towards mutual support in the family, household interests in migration are

[16] Rephrased statement of interviewees P2F and P5M.

likely to gain influence in the course of concrete migration decision-making.

This said, the students' current migration projects present as individual biographic strategies rather than livelihood strategies of a family or household: high aspirations on personal and professional development in their combination with the weight of family reciprocity turn the attention to appealing opportunities abroad. As the discussion has exposed, those individual approaches to migration remain rooted in the students' family contexts: firstly, they are developed within the frame of anticipated family expectations and life scripts of reciprocity; secondly the concept of migration as step towards self-empowerment and independence explains only in the light of a strong family influence on the life course. Thus, what presents as an individual migration project is partly an individual response to family-related living conditions.

Where gendered expectations to care are not interfering, this does not translate into a restrictive factor for the personal migration outlook, as the students tend to take a positive attitude towards the malleability of distance in family relations - at least under the conditions of return. This attitude characterizes them generally speaking as "*reluctant distant thinkers*" (Mason 1999 quoted in Baldassar, Vellekoop Baldock and Wilding 2007: 217) who feel able to realize their personal temporary migration projects in accordance with their familial environment. Long-term effects of temporary migration on families left behind are expected to be overwhelmingly positive (economic improvements e.g. in housing, education- and health care access) as long as migrants' would maintain in contact with their families and support them economically (see Annex Table 1).

## The Personal Development Project

The students' images about empowerment and self-determination by means of migration make reference to aims of personal development, expressing individualist self-identities which shape the character of their life plans with claims towards personal entitlements and ownership of biographic decision-making. Their desire for personal development manifests most concretely in a personal agenda of self-actualisation driven by the hunger for individualized modern lifestyles and the privileges of lifestyle choice they associate with life in *Western* societies. Their expectancy of lifestyles abroad comprises a social dimension related to tolerance towards women with liberal lifestyles and socializing with people from other cultures, and a material dimension of access to Internet technology, public infrastructure, leisure time activities and tourism. The students' desires to experience different lifestyles through migration intertwine with reflexive and globalized self-identities. Their ideas of lifestyle choices abroad reveal a symbolic value of reflexivity and allow a critical reflection of the discourse on lifestyle migration.

The treated biographic projects and ideas on professional development and the role of family attachment for the future life have already disclosed a fundamental conviction about the personal entitlement to develop individual future perspectives and adopt strategic choices in order to pursue personal projects throughout the life course. Valuing personal assertiveness, refusing marriage or seeking personal savings and professional authority, as well as last but not least individually designed and pushed migration plans reflect visions of lifestyles promoting individual *ownership* of the future life. Such visions settle individual choice as a common value of life scripts and self-identities in the sense of an individualization of the life plan. According to Giddens (1991), the latter requires essentially an awareness of individual options and choices of particular self-identities and lifestyles.

### *Lifestyle Choice*

To capture the important role of lifestyle in late-modern individuals' reflexive self-identity projects, Featherstone, referring to Giddens, has proposed to approach lifestyle needs as a material and non-material way to design and express the reflexive self beyond a socially determined identity script:

"Rather than unreflexively adopting a lifestyle, through tradition or habit, the new heroes [...] make lifestyle a life project and display their individuality and sense of style in the particularity of the assemblage of goods, clothes, practices, experiences, appearance and bodily dispositions they design together into a lifestyle." (Featherstone 1987: 59)

A broader lifestyle dimension of migration as an assemblage of body, consume and experience in the sense of Featherstone surfaces in the students' description of the transition or the *rite of passage* (see p. 15) that migrant nurses allegedly undergo:

"They come back changed, modernised, rich, their body looks nice and attractive"; and "they come here looking beautiful, rich and very educated." (Written statements of WS3 and WS5)

Self-actualisation as component of the personal transition associated with migration is partly conceptualized as a matter of space and environment, linking ideas of spatial and social mobility:

"Participant 2F: I think, I can develop, there can be that personal development when I go there. [...] It can be exciting, it can be an achievement, personal achievement, ya. Because like, within myself, apart from the basic needs that I want in my life, there is also self-actualization. Of which one of them is to go abroad and see those different places. [...][Self-actualization] is like to be satisfied to achieve what I wanted. Like to not necessarily having the material part of things but just be at a place where I've always dreamed of to be. Not necessarily maybe getting some more or a lot of money, whatsoever. But just having that quality life that I've always wanted to be in." (Interview P2F: 14)

"Participant 5M: [...] and also socializing with people there: I would like to specialize with people who live in the UK, I would like to socialize with people who live in the UK so that I can see life at another perspective of life, at another angle, see what happens there comparing with what happens here in Malawi. That way I will have a broader perspective of what life is." (Interview P5M: 6)

Lifestyle choice, approached as a matter of placing oneself in a social and physical setting by choice, is portrayed as a privilege that allows imagining and experiencing the *social space* of reference as an individually definable and expandable one. Beyond the students' expectations to make specific lifestyle experiences abroad, Featherstone's idea of *lifestyle choice* emerged as a common aspect of the students' migration intentions. The concept of "*reflexive habitus*" (Sweetman 2003: 537), meaning that habitus is not necessarily constituted by *what* is chosen but may as well be shaped by the self-perception and entitlement to make *reflexive choice* itself, bears an interesting analytic perspective on these aspirations and images[17]: entitlements of reflexive choice appear relevant to the globalized habitus definition of the young nursing elite, taking into account the common recognition that migration would increase the range of available choices on life and lifestyles.

Lifestyle affinity as a pattern of social belonging reveals at the same time as a generational matter, bringing about a new importance of lifestyle issues and a related attractiveness of migration among Malawian middleclass youth:

"[...] I have noted for me that this generation, in our nation we are even giving more worth to questions of lifestyle. It is a difference from a few years ago. So our generations we are sort of copying with the *Western* cultures, as in terms of technology, lifestyle and all that stuff. Now: as she (P22F) has put it: 15 years ago we would not go drive at night for a cinema. But now you go around at night, sitting around in town, after midnight, driving. So that kind of lifestyle that is typical to us can motivate some people to go [abroad] for that. Saying that's the way I want my life." (WS 3, P23M: 16)

The reasoning of P23M points to a new importance of lifestyle activities in the definition of and requirement for social membership to the young generation of Malawian peers. The latter is associated with the perception that the new way of life is a practice of relating to and acquiring admission to globalization, growing upon and reinforcing the social ties to *Western cultures* and shaping a collective self-identity, constructing itself as transnational, *Western* and modern. P5M's above cited motivation to study abroad

---

17 Sweetman (2003) develops this concept in a different context, with reference to particularly reflexive self-identities in late modern societies. Yet, it appears fruitful to this analysis as well, as it captures Giddens' argument of individualized self-identities and life plans and brings it into one picture with Bourdieu's argument about the influence of habitus and status requirements on professional and social aspirations and choices.

inscribes partly into this lifestyle trend of the educated Malawian youth as it allows participating in an international network of the highly skilled elite, to which the students feel attached by the shared *Western* professional curriculum of nursing, as well as wider habitus and lifestyle aspirations. Migration is likely to gain further symbolic value as a privilege to access lifestyle choice and global social membership in the current political climate of migration regimes increasingly restricting the choice of youth from African countries to leave.

### *Lifestyle Dimensions of the Migration Project*

Tracing in the following the concrete dimensions of the attractiveness of lifestyles abroad and the specific lifestyle issues in the students' migration projects, different, partly ambiguously evaluated aspects reveal. To several students, lifestyle has an essentially material meaning, related to goods like good food, advanced technology or improved health care (written statements), pointing to a reasoning that associates lifestyle with high standard of living as an effect of higher income:

> "Having money, it can change your life. Because if you have enough money, not necessarily enough, but then you have all this money that you can help yourself with and that you can even help your relatives although they are here. So thereby you might choose, maybe one day, I still want to go in town, or have good things and stuff. It's still changing your lifestyle- even whilst you have your responsibilities for you families here. Somehow the lifestyle will still be fortunate with the better standards of living. […] It becomes all miserable when it comes to the point where you're so tired at the end of the month. You're getting the bills; somebody is coming along, school fees and that and this and that. And then sometimes you don't even eat properly, you don't even dress up as if you were good-looking - it becomes stressing." (WS 5, P35F: 11)

Within the already tackled tension between family-relatedness and individualization of the life script, the attribution of money and time to lifestyle must be considered an exclusive luxury, hardly attainable with a nurses' income in Malawi and under the conditions of financial responsibility for family members.

Beyond the dimension of material consume of lifestyles, *Western* societies, imagined as a world of liberal values and lifestyle plurality, are particularly attractive to students with a strong self-identity of a *reformer* (see Table 6, p. 68). Their high commitment to the individual career development is mirrored in the personal sphere by an agenda of experiencing self-actualisation, diverse emancipatory lifestyle freedoms, social innovation, as well as a high degree of personal independence.

Single female nursing students in this cluster, for whom gendered lifestyle choices (such as single life) are an essential factor of self-identity and life planning, evaluate the lifestyle impact of migration against female lifestyle patterns accessible and sanctioned in Malawi. Their gender-related future visions of migration relate to lifestyles as forms of constructing and expressing individuality through modern partnership models including role-switching and independent accountancy, or the avoidance of marriage - aspects already tackled in former chapters. The consumption of entertainment with friends as a single woman falls into the same realm:

> "Maybe, for example, someone likes going out[*]. Here in Malawi that would be this weekend you go with these people, the other weekend you go out with these other people - people will regard you as a prostitute. But maybe out there in UK people can go out without a name being attached to them. So you can say I will go, just to enjoy your life." [*she did, as the interview revealed] (WS 5, P36F: 10-11)

> "On my personal thing: It's all about having that free life because, for me, I haven't had that free life because of our culture. You have to be, people call you names, so people call you: `Uh, that girl is a prostitute, that girl is uff´- those things, just because of our culture." (Interview P36F: 13-14)

In the case of P36F, access to liberal lifestyle environments as a single woman emerges as a decisive aspect in the preference for a life abroad. The need for financial resources for the personal and family demands and her conflict with local gender roles constitute her main motivations to leave. Her story exposes the potential weight of vague ideas of lifestyle empowerment through migration, as she otherwise feels strongly attached to bedside nursing in Malawi and could imagine to work as a community nurse in a rural area, under the condition of entertainment in a town area being accessible to her.

In the small group of study participants who approach migration positively and design temporally open migration projects, the prospect to access new lifestyles and broaden the personal and professional perspective is a common biographic aspiration to migrate. Previous studies on Malawian nurses' migration intentions have already highlighted this basic lifestyle dimension of migration and non-return decisions (Grigulis 2010).

On the contrary, students characterized as *Care-givers* (see Table 6, p. 68), whose individual lifestyles follow conservative biographic priorities of marriage and settlement in Malawi, either neglect or problematize lifestyle issues of their migration project, though they acknowledge the availability of personal development opportunities linked to further education, economic independence and social capital (e.g. Interview P27F and P14M). In this regard, some students expect to be hindered in their personal development by experiences of violence and xenophobia as well as challenges to adapt to a new and more liberal social environment.[18] In particular with regard to the separation from family members the impact of migration for the personal development project was evaluated as ambiguous, torn between appreciating higher independence and fearing the psychological challenges of a disconcerting lonely life far from home (e.g. Interview P31F and P14M). Students with a strong desire to follow religious practices furthermore worried about religious restrictions.

### *Lifestyle Migration from the Global South?*

Whereas the above analysis has pointed clearly to the importance of lifestyle motivations for Malawian nurses' migration projects, the academic discourse on lifestyle migration tends to ignore the impact of lifestyle questions on the South-North migration of the highly skilled. Benson and O'Reilly, giving a review of the literature on lifestyle migration, regard it

---

[18] E.g. when watching an American movie together, some female students expressed disgust when being exposed to kissing and touching couples.

„[...] as specifically to the relative economic privilege of individuals in the developed world, the reflexivity evident in post-/late modernity, the construction of particular places as offering alternative lifestyles, and a more general ease (or freedom) of movement. […] The search for a better way of life while held in common with other migrants such as refugees and asylum seekers, here implies something distinct, connoting a particular lifestyle choice specific to individuals of the developed world.“ (Benson and O'Reilly 2009: 620)

In arguing that the privilege of lifestyle choices in the late-modern, developed world would define lifestyle migration as a mobility among the wealthy *Western* elite only, they overlook the impact of globalization on the life concepts of individuals in less prosperous regions and the attractiveness of transnationally circulating social images about the privileged *West* as a world of a appealing lifestyles. Even if lifestyle migration is a product of the specific conditions of late-modernity, it has considerable repercussions in countries of the *Global South*: images about *Western* lifestyle worlds, promising superior life standard, lifestyle plurality and the luxury of accessing lifestyle activities, are an essential part of the young nursing graduates' desire to leave. Transnational dynamics, such as the social remittances of those coming back *changed, rich, beautiful and educated* (see p. 126), can easily establish a symbolic value of lifestyle migration in home societies in the *Global South*. Beyond this, the globalized universe of the media nurtures visions of the lifestyle world of health workers overseas, as highlighted by the comment of a Lebanese medical student in a study on migration intentions: "*By thinking of medicine, you immediately think of ''ER'' and ''Chicago Hope. It's like everything is registered in your unconsciousness'* ' (Akl et al. 2007: 1281). Playing in US hospital settings, the relationships and lifestyle debates of the upper class of prestigious American health professionals are situated in the heart of these soap operas. Also in the Malawian nursing college it was common to watch American movies during the lunch break.

While the attraction towards alternative lifestyles and individual lifestyle choice is frequent, with few exceptions it does not lead to long-term migration projects. Instead, the time abroad is envisaged as a biographic period to explore and enjoy new lifestyles and access a different standard of living. The imagination about return inherits the expectation to have sufficient cultural and economic capital to ease the burden of obligations towards the family and allow fulfilling ones' material lifestyle aspirations back in Malawi.

This situation does not apply to women for whom lifestyle connects strongly with self-development and gender-related empowerment issues: the tangly connection between lifestyle choice, modern lifestyles and empowerment ties their aspirations towards self-determination and equality to a life in the imagined social space of a *Western* country. Even where personal savings would preserve economic independence, these conditions to realize the personal life script are not transferable to Malawi. However, none of these women attempts to draw a clear cut between life before and after migration, as typical among lifestyle-migrants from the Global North (Benson and O'Reilly 2009). None of the women anticipated confronting negative reputation in Malawi due to her exposure to modern lifestyles abroad, a situation found to complicate e.g. the return of women migrants from Bangladesh (Dannecker 2005). Instead, these young women combine striving to experience independent lifestyles abroad with maintaining family relations and ties of solidarity; they introduce spatial distance to protect their social and family bonds as well as their personal integrity, as has been discussed in depth regarding the family orientation of the life plan.

## Religious Guidance

As Christianity presents with 82,7% of the population the major religion in Malawi (NSO 2009), all interviewed students are affiliates of Christian churches. They belong to different groups of Christians, ranging from Catholics, over Presbyterians and a variety of Pentecostal churches to Jehovah's witnesses.[19] Pentecostal

[19] The specific church membership was tackled in seven out of the ten interviews.

churches such as Assemblies of God, Bible Believers, and Holy Ghost and Evangelism ministry were dominant in this subgroup. The broad spectrum of different affiliations in particular to Pentecostal churches reflects the fast growth of these churches and ministries in Malawi (Englund 2004; Forster 1997).

The interviews and observations reveal that religious practice, next to family advice, constitutes a central guideline of the biographic project and a superior frame of reference of future life imagination. Many students thematize praying as an important practice when making decisions for their lives. Furthermore, praying is perceived as a major factor of encouragement: towards hard work, particularly in education, towards moral maturity and when coping with disappointments of the life plan, e.g. in the case of deviations of the career choice towards nursing.

The students express deep confidence that their God, who would guide and bless them for their efforts, would direct their life to the good. This does however not translate into a worldview of divine providence and collective planning determining the future life and contradicting individual ownership of the life course.[20] For several students spiritual development and worship present as separate angle of the future life plan, while others simply regard religion as a permanent guidance through every day life.

Though religious life projects are not at the forefront of the nursing students' reasoning about migration, the strong importance of religion in their scripts of life raises the question to what extend religious perceptions and experiences interact with their aspiration to migrate. Research on religion and migration has highlighted the global and cosmopolitan dimensions of Christian religious organizations and spiritualties, concluding: "*religion is a global societal system as transnational in its operation as the economy or the nation-state*" (Levitt 2003: 848). Four dimensions of African Christianities' global links are considered as relevant to the context of this study and will be focused upon in this chapter.

---

[20] If, on the contrary, divine providence or collective planning had been regarded as determinant of future life, the applied research approach to an individual life plan would very likely have been rejected.

The first aspect concerns the historical linkages of African churches to European and North American ones, established and maintained through missionary activities of migrants, crusaders and colonizers: In the case of Malawi, it was the Scotland-based Livingstonia mission that initiated the era of European invasion and the international colonial ties of religious communities caused a tensioned relation between religion and the project of sovereign national development of the Banda regime (Forster 1997). Since then, mission Christianity has been shaping and influencing locally founded churches decidedly (Englund 2003).

Grigulis (2010) points to an eventual importance of historical religious ties in the choice of destination countries among Malawian overseas nurses, as her interviewees often lived in Scotland and belonged to churches originating from Scotland. Though the link to Scottish churches did not reflect in the reports of the nursing students I interviewed, freedom of worship and the availability of religious services were considered as an important issue for members of the church of Jehovah's witnesses when contemplating possible destinations:

> "[…] before I would go abroad I would consider some other issues like religion. To say, if I would be at a certain campus how long would I need to be traveling to my church and back? How much time would I need to devote to my studies? And see how that affects my religious part and so forth. And then I would also consider: Is it accepted in that particular area, because there are some lands, where Jehovah's witnesses are not allowed to practice their faith. So I would also consider those things: If there is no problem with that, then I would go." (Interview P31F: 15)

Her awareness and alertness about religious restrictions in other countries might be particular to members of her religious community, due to its historical experiences of oppression and persecution in Malawi, particularly during the long era of president Banda, as well as in many other countries, e.g. South Africa and several European countries (Forster 1997, Penton 1999). Such concerns were not expressed among members of other Christian groups, which could be explained with regard to the global networks of European and African Christianities, making spiritual services available in most global metropoles and thus weakening the historical religious links to specific destinations (Vásquez 2009). In spite of that, none of the students mentioned to consider leaving for a Muslim country though e.g. Saudi Arabia is a major global destination of nurse migration. This may be regarded as a hint at the implicit importance of shared religious self- and social identities in the choice of destination, found among migrants from Muslim countries as well (Dannecker 2005).

The second aspect regards the spiritual ideas of global membership that establish a cosmopolitan sense of belonging, alleviating the essentially local meaning of *homeness* that attaches people to their surrounding. As has been argued by Englund (2004) for Pentecostal Christianities in Malawi, the Christian religious idea of being in the evil material word, as compared to being in the spiritual space of encounter with God, builds an idea of spiritual *homeness* that transcends local belonging. At the same time, a global portability of religious ties can be established via practices of public worship that localize religious spirituality in specific spirits and material objects, establishing experiences of the "*dialectic between the materialisation of the spirit and spiritualisation of the material at various spatio-temporal scales*" (Vásquez 2009: 280).

Though these patterns of global spiritual belonging do not reflect directly in the findings of this research, a global reference of spirituality emerges in women nurses' perception of their professional mission as a universal one (see p. 93). Approaching their involuntary career deviation into nursing as a blessing of the Holy Ghost to serve God's mission of care for any human alike, their future professional vocation is dedicated to a global mission of care that transcends the attachment to a particular place. The religious self-identity inscribes here into the transnational professional habitus of the students and establishes a fundamental legitimacy of the intention to migrate, "*using religion to create an alternative allegiance of belonging*" (Levitt 2003: 851) and meaning (ibid.). Levitt writes this describing the transnational practices of migrants and stating that such materially "*unobservable dimensions of religious life*" (ibid.) tend to be undervalued in transnational studies, while they constitute an important, identity-relevant practice of migrants and migrant communities.

The third dynamic of interest concerns the *symbolic ties* (Faist 1998) establishing between community members back home and abroad as a result of transnational activities and social identities that create upon shared religious affiliations. As has been shown for Ghanaian members of Pentecostal churches, their imagination of the religious community extends to a global dimension, promising the individual membership in a worldwide community of believers. This imagination serves as a powerful point of reference for the individual religious self-identity formation and anchors the self as a global, rather than a local subject (van Dijk 2002).

Such religious conceptions of the self are likely to find fertile ground in the students and nourish their aspirations towards membership to a global community. Though frequent praying and ministry as well as spiritual development were outlined in several cases as important angles of the future life, caveats to leave a local congregation to go abroad were absent in the students' accounts, which may be read as a hint that they hold globalized conceptions of their religious community of reference. Links to local congregations can however also generate transnational religious practices of migrant members, including financial contributions, long-distance guidance or home visits (Levitt 2003). Mkwinda-Nyasulu and Chilemba (2007) have pointed to the relevance of such religiously mediated transnationalism in Malawi regarding the diaspora engagement of overseas professionals in the Seventh Day Adventist church in the USA, who run the "Operation Reach Back".

Another aspect of a transnational constructions of religious identity can be perceived among Pentecostals in West Africa, where the teaching of local churches engages strongly in the promotion of migration, up to the promise of spiritual and material service for the realization of transnational life projects and migration plans, as well as for the mission of social modernization and individualization modelled to allegedly *Western* values (van Diyk 2002; Hunt 2002). Though none of the students pointed directly to such church services, several stated that they would consult a priest when making a migration decision (Quest.). Of interest is also the story of P25F discussed earlier (see p. 107): she makes reference to the influence of encounters with male international visitors to her father's Pentecostal ministry, who shaped her idea of finding an appropriate liberally-thinking husband abroad. As her case suggests, globally active religious communities in Malawi may also have an impact on the local ideas about the benefits of migration and the values of *Western* societies, if transnational spaces of intercultural exposure are created within the local congregation.

Fourthly, the coexistence of highly individualist and highly religious self-identities in the students' life stories indicates that they stand in a positive relationship (e.g. Interviews P25F, P2F and P36F). Beyond the direct global linkages between religion and migration explored ahead, the trend of Pentecostal churches to promote independent and self-determined life scripts is therefore relevant to our context, as it reflects closely the students' self-identities, their career orientation and aspiration to pursue self-determined biographic projects.

> "[…] [T]he doctrines expressed [by Pentecostal Christianities in West Africa] move away from the sectarian and millenarian focus of traditional black Pentecostalism and have come to embrace some of the core values of *Western* society: materialism, success, careerism and human potential. The teachings, values and overarching ethos of these black Pentecostal churches with their emphasis on equality of opportunity, alongside free choice, also encourage members to regard themselves as authors of their own identity and biographies, and to constantly reflect upon themselves in order to shape their futures rather than engendering a feeling of resignation and fatalism." (Hunt 2002: 165)

These religious advices address the ambivalences between divine determination and familial obligations of reciprocity on the one hand, attempts towards individual self-determination and reflexive self-identities on the other hand: Pentecostal churches promote a conjugal rather than an extended family model, providing an ethical framework to bring kinship obligations under the individual members' supervision while contesting family and traditional authority, which become associated with backwardness and ignorance (van Dijk 2002). This reflects closely the family orientation of the students' life plans. The Pentecostal family image is characterized by a strong ambivalence between family as an important emotional bound and an evil source of domination, as it also emerges in statements of P36F who complains having to live the life of her parents (see p. 115). Such reasoning supports the students' migration intentions driven by self-empowerment, individual professional advancement and personal development.

At the same time, the religiously constructed sense of individuality carries an ambiguous concept of individualism that should not be mistaken for a liberal approach to self-determination in the terms of Giddens. Instead, the idea and habitus of individual self-determination stand under strict doctrines of religious ethics and leaders' authority (van Dijk 2002), consecrating subjectivity to a higher power, as Englund (2003) observes for the Malawian context. Nonetheless, charismatic Christianities promoting the transmission of such identity concepts to (religious) communities establish pro-migratory attitudes and conditions (van Dijk 2002): their religious underpinnings for values of individualism and modernity help creating a delocalized and globalized habitus that strengthens the amalgamation of migration and individualization discernible also in the students' different life projects.

This religiously guided discourse of individuality and migration, the global mission of nursing as well as the transnational linkages of African Christianities are to be considered as religious elements of the broader social dynamics of globalisation in Malawi, that shape pro-migratory attitudes among nursing students. As religious advices and prayers are quotidian practices to gain moral guidance for life decisions, pro-migratory religious ethics and practices are likely to strengthen the viability of the individual migration intention subtly but fundamentally.

## The Social and Socioeconomic Project

The students' life projects of social and socioeconomic development commingle social status ambitions, ideas of social change and multiple affiliations to transnationally as well as a locally defined communities. A personal and moral attachment, resulting in the will to make a social contribution to 'their' country or for 'their' people, forms part of the migration and return ideas in most students' life plans. Guided by elite self-identities of not wanting to be an *"average person"* (Interview P5M: 7), most students express high expectations of status mobility in Malawi, including the improvement of their job position, their economic position, social recognition and influence. Those are linked to ideas of becoming actors of '*development*' in their home society, countering the social image of migrant nurses abandoning their people.

The students' mostly temporary migration projects establish transnational social identities evolving in the interplay between global references in their habitus and local attachment as well as status aspirations *back home*[21]. This interplay places their personal migration projects within the frame of the public expectations they confront in Malawi: relating their migration plans to social discourses of *brain drain*, *brain gain* and *development,* they design social and socioeconomic biographic projects through which they acquire important justifications for their aspirations to go abroad. Parallel to local attachment, their biographic ambitions are directed towards participation in the global community of the highly skilled. This social biographic project displays in references to a globalized habitus based in international exposure and transnational practices as pathways to expertise and status.

### *Going Global & Turning Homewards*

As has been argued by Bauman, social perceptions in a globalized world tend to establish a hierarchic antithesis between the global and the local sphere:

"Today's existence is stretched along the hierarchy of the global and the

---

[21] See Footnote 9 (p.15) for the terminology of *home*.

local, with global freedom of movement signalling social promotion, advancement and success, and immobility exuding the repugnant odour of defeat, failed life and being left behind." (Bauman 1998: 121)

„Increasingly, globality and locality acquire the character of contrary values – […] placed in the very centre of life dreams, nightmares and struggles. […] Freedom came to mean above all freedom of choice, and choice has acquired, conspicuously, a spatial dimension." (Bauman 2000: 216)

Bauman regards this hierarchy of values as characteristic for the influence of globalization on migrants' perspectives as well as for the establishing of migration as a socially sanctioned *rite of passage* (see p. 15). Students' arguments about the potential to advance socially and develop their home country through migration reflect their adherence to hierarchical ideas about the *global* over the *local*[22]. Regarding the first aspect of advancing socially, their statements reveal the expectation that migration would open chances to acquire particular social capital and socially embodied cultural capital by way of international exposure to inspiring academic environments:

"Participant27F: […] I can profit from that, because going abroad you meet different people, you make some connections and some people can also help you develop in life. [...] Most of the times, people get matured in terms of knowledge due to exposure to different personalities and different people. Ok, I can give an example of somebody who has not been to college and somebody who has been to college: The knowledge status differs. Even if the other one is a genius (laughing) in terms of being in class, but exposure to different people also helps you in knowledge development." (Interview P27F: 13)

"Participant25F: I can't just say, it's something that will come as an opportunity, but it's something in my plan to say: At some point in time I will need to go out. [...] I can't say it's good to do everything in Malawi [...]. It's different and it's good to have an experience, not just because it's the same thing they are doing, teaching. No, just by the change of environment, having different people and everything it makes you learn.

[22] Italic font is used in the following to demarcate the words "global" and "local" when used in the sense of Baumann.

[…] So I feel not just for the sake of my education or for the sake of me having experience or working outside for maybe some years but then even as in personally I can learn something." (Interview P25F: 10-11)

According to these accounts, migration as a biographical project to develop socially is closely attached to the personal hunt for knowledge, skills and maturation (to embody cultural capital), as well as for helpful networks (social capital). At the same time, the remark of P25F that *'it's the same thing they are doing'* makes clear that she regards herself as equally well trained to British nurses and entitled to participate in the imagined privileged environment of an international nursing elite. Having studied the *ideal nursing* of the British curriculum (see p. 83-85) acts as a proof of belonging where this knowledge can be applied and enhanced. The students hope to be received as equal members to a global academic community of equally trained nurses, which they expect offering more fertile cultures of learning (in particular close interaction with and appreciative supervision by teachers) as well as favourable conditions of practice (e.g. well equipped hospitals).

Considering here the students' social identity as Malawi's academic elite (see p. 78-79; 83-85) and new lifestyle-oriented generation (see p. 127-28), on a more abstract level a globalized social peer-identity takes shape, which may be characterized as an imagined global community of a *Western,* personally and professionally developing academic elite. It links local and global spheres of references into a transnational habitus and attributes to the migration experience a value in itself, as compared to the instrumental value of expected outcomes of migration such as personal savings or an academic title.

To trace manifestations of this transnational habitus, transnational practices in the students' social peer environment of academic nurses in Malawi are relevant, where role models often possess international experience, which they transfer: UNIMA lecturers are generally supposed to hold Master or PHD titles, usually requiring a stage of studies abroad. While lack of highly qualified professionals in the country has hindered UNIMA from reinforcing this principle strictly (UNIMA 2010), international experience was found to be normality among students' academic role models in the campus environment:

"Participant2F: When she went there and she stayed there for three months, at her friend's place, whilst doing some other studies. And then she went to the hospital directly. [...] I met her here [in the nursing college]. When I was in first year, she was here pursuing her midwifery. So we used to be good friends! Yeah! That's where I got to know much about her: here.

Researcher: Mhm. And do you think she would invite you? Would she try to help you if you went abroad?

Participant2F: Yeah! That's what she has been telling me (laughing), yeah, because she went to the UK, because she had a friend here at Kamuzu College of Nursing. She told me that when she was here, at KCN, in her first year, she had a friend who was also pursuing a certificate in midwifery. So she was like: `I also want to do the same thing that I was done by the other person. So [...] she wanted to give back the favour that she was done by the other person, yeah. (Laughing)" (Interview P2F: 18)

Such practices institute a *culture of migration* that nourishes *global* orientations and a habitus of mobility aspirations in the students' social peer environment. It establishes transnational social bonds between students at KCN, as the idea of reciprocity translates into a commitment to support the migration prospects of following generations.

At the same time, this contextualization of young nursing academics' migration projects indicates that they might seek migration more in their social role as university graduates than in their professional context as nurses: considering firstly that Malawi's last population census 2008 revealed a high and continuously increasing rate of international migration for study purposes[23], secondly

[23] The census claims portraying non-return migration, which is naturally higher in very recent years, when temporary and non-return migrants are not distinguishable. However, the data depicts clearly that since 2002 a substantial and increasing number of young people leave Malawi to seek further studies. It is likely that this trend goes back to university degree holders and professionals

that nursing students' partners were also generally seeking to migrate for further studies, and thirdly that the academic environment on other campuses bears similar international linkages, the assumption is fair that not specifically nursing students but the young generation of Malawian academics in general nurture a *culture of migration* establishing foreign degrees and international exposure as part of a globalized academic habitus. Regarding academic nurses in Malawi, this raises the question whether restrictive migration regimes could lead to a negative reputation of nursing among prospective students and hinder the recruitment into the profession in the medium term.

Extending these observations beyond the Malawian context, it seems important to recognize that the students' symbolic valuing of global academic environments mirrors the narratives of mobility among international students from developed countries closely. Hinting at the development of a common, globalized habitus of international mobility in the class of privileged academics from countries in the Global North as well as the *Global South*, this supports the observations of Findlay et al. (2012) that

> "[…] migrating to learn may be part of the process of learning to migrate. The suggestion here is that [international] student mobility is not simply a subset of youth mobility culture, but part of a wider set of mobility cultures linked to a person's outlook on their entire life-course (Brooks and Everett 2008)." (Ibid.: 122)

> "It appears that a 'world-class' education for some is embedded in a mobility culture that attaches symbolic capital to the very performance of international living […]." (Ibid.: 128)

The above discussion of students' social linkage to the global academic elite would have suggested a future design guided by ideas of global mobility. To the contrary, their discourse of return as essential element of future life leads to a more complicated picture: on the level of the life plan, *global* perspectives are being integrated with a biographic appreciation of going *home*.

---

with internationally recognized qualifications in particular, who are granted access to tertiary education abroad.

The students' ideas of return stands in the context of concerns about social rejection abroad, caused by xenophobia, discrimination and violence, which they name as most important challenges for migrants, in particular in South Africa. The focus of such negative images on South Africa may be explained by the high media presence of anti-immigrant riots there, as well as by a vivid social memory of the historical experiences of Malawian migrants in the colonial economy and in Apartheid South Africa (see p. 26-27). Also in other destinations, several students anticipate racism and violence to complicate Malawian overseas nurses' participation, safety and joyfulness in social life, shaping reluctance towards opportunities of general social membership abroad and a reasoning why return would be an imperative to find a happy future (WS 1; WS 2). In contrast, several students' proudly stated that their country had never seen a war, pointing to high levels of security and a culture of peacefulness, regarded as benefits of a life in Malawi that could easily be lost in other countries:

> "There you cannot live the life you always wanted. As for me, I love my country and I've realized it's a peaceful country and it is very different what people are experiencing in these other countries." (WS 4, P25F: 15)

As is noticeable in this statement as well, far most students express a strong social identification with their home community, as they integrate migration into life plans that fundamentally orient towards a future in the Malawian society. The students' representations of a promising, happy future in Malawi articulate in the saying "*home is home, home is best*" (WS 4, P32F: 14), as well as in various confessions of emotional attachment.

> "And you go for some years and then you come back, because when you go there you miss your relatives, your family. You may have a lot of money in your pocket, [...] you may have a good life, but social contact with your relatives is very important." (WS 2, P15M: 12)

This emotional factor combines for most students with a strongly status-related one. It entangles expectations towards personal development abroad with expectations that this development would increase the personal status in Malawi, to the extent that the future life in the aftermath of migration would confer to the living standards of an elite member of society. This connection has already been discussed regarding the students' professional life projects, within which migration is sought to improve the occupational respectively social status as an academic nurse in Malawi to a level of distinction (see p. 77-78; 85-88).

The aspiration to generate economic wealth by means of migration is part of this reasoning:

"And also when you are there and you have money, they wouldn't recognize you, because everybody has money. Everybody is driving like a pushy car. You come back here with a pushy car and everybody will be looking at you." (WS 2, P11F: 12)

"So you go for some time, you make money, you upgrade your academia, you come back and get an important position." (WS 2, P15M: 12)

As these statements of P11F and P15M indicate, the value of resources produced in the course of migration tends to be evaluated with respect to the home, not the destination country: *back home*, the cultural, social, economic and symbolic capitals accumulated abroad are thought to guarantee privileged income perspectives, the hoarded personal savings to translate directly into social status. This contextualizes economic reasons to migrate in a broader life-course perspective.

Applying Bourdieu's (1986) theory about the different conversion rates of capitals to this situation, the students' migration projects explain as strategies to convert their advanced cultural, social and economic capital at a particularly high rate because it possesses a value of scarcity in Malawi. The enhanced value of these capitals is thought to assure access to ever more social and cultural capital, translating into high economic capital and ultimately into the satisfaction of occupational, economic and social status aspirations as members of the educated Malawian elite. In this context, a high instrumental value of migration becomes evident.

While most study participants join the discourse of *home is best,* a few presume persistent local gender roles and professional hierarchies to build overwhelming barriers for their social status mobility in Malawi, evaluating their social perspectives abroad as more rewarding, also in the long term. These participants assume better chances of professional status mobility based on a higher social appreciation for nurses abroad (WS 1), or, in the case of female students, suppose that liberal and plural societies abroad would allow them higher social participation and respect as single or independent women (WS 5; Interview P36F).

### *Migration for Empowerment & Development*

Ideas of migration-for-empowerment have been revealing in the context of different life projects explored already. The intention to migrate in search of global opportunities and entitlements inherits a g*lobal* emancipatory idea, which characterizes the students as global political subjects in the sense of Giddens. He describes "*emancipatory politics*" (Giddens 1995: 7 and 1991) as a political quarrel for life chances, threatened by socioeconomic inequalities in the global arena. Giddens' concept of emancipatory politics only applies partially to our context, as the nursing students represent a socioeconomically privileged group in their local context and as notions of migration as a protest against the global distribution of resources do not express directly in their reasoning. The concept appertains nonetheless to the status struggle of nurses in the local hospital hierarchy: in this context, the students pursue migration as a *vote with their feet*, protesting against political institutions and occupational conditions which to their mind ignore their interests and necessities. Next to this, migration to escape and transform restrictive gender roles forms part of a social project of emancipative politics. Reflecting the turn from emancipative to *life politics* (ibid.), which Giddens identifies as characteristic of the postmodern world, the students' ways of asserting claims take the form of biographic strategies of self-actualization, implicitly politicizing life decisions that affect their self-identities. Gender has become central to *life politics, as* politics going back to the dialectic intrusion between the global and local sphere in the reflexive projects of self and society in a context of globalisation and late modernity:

"Women across the world now stake a claim to forms of autonomy previously denied or unavailable to them. [...] [H]owever, that claim to autonomy intrudes deeply into the domain of life politics, for it raises issues to do with the very definition of what it is to be a woman, and therefore a man, in detraditionalizing societies and cultures." (Giddens 1995: 11)

Women nurses' strategies of migration and empowerment inscribe into this context as they seek to experience through migration an environment of individual, emancipatory lifestyles and lifestyle choices that is essential to their self and peer-groups' identity, as well as their aspired way of independent living *back home*. This connection reveals most pronounced in the case of P32F, who envisages that her emancipatory migration project would equip her economically to live in Malawi in disaccord with traditional gender roles and resisting gendered lifestyle restrictions (Interview P32F).

This *life political* aspect of the students' migration intentions brings global entitlements and social remittances together: it draws upon elite self- and social-identities, embracing claims of entitlements to *global* experiences on the one hand, to the transformation of *local* conditions in Malawi on the other hand. It circumscribes transnational fields, sought to liberate from the curtailment of the public life course for Malawian's educated youth, to design paths of social development back home, as well as to newly encounter with the local social context as an emancipated and renewed subject. The recurrent positive symbolic connotations of migrants coming back beautiful, modernized and changed (see p. 126) suggests a higher social tolerance towards diverging lifestyles and behaviours of returnees, i.e. a different fundament to bring individualized lifestyles and choices of (gendered) identity into agreement with aspirations towards prestige in the local society.

The students' elitist mission of distinctive self-development, located exclusively in the social context of a developed world, conceptualizes *Western* countries and the UK in particular as a *global* social space and reservoir of what is *locally* inaccessible. It embeds the individual migration intentions in the global conditions of structural inequalities. Beyond this, it situates the students' mindsets within a (post)colonial, bipolar discourse about the developed versus the developing world. It established an antithetical and hierarchical mental geography of the *global* vs. the *local*, development vs. stagnation and decline in the terms of Bauman (see p. 140).

In the following discussion, the students' discourse on migration and development will be scrutinized, situating the personal migration projects within the global debate on *brain gain* and the local discourse on *brain drain.* As Nieswand (2011) elaborates, positive linkages of migration and (trans)national attachment to development in the home society have been transforming the political dialogue on South-North migration in many destination countries, diaspora communities and African countries of origin throughout the past decade. The Malawian political discourse on nurse migration does not seem to have incorporated this positive point of view on migration so far, as political documents and discussions tackle migration of skilled professionals and nurse migration in particular unanimously as problem or challenge (Durevall and Mussa 2010; Muula 2006b).

The strong presence of positive views on the development potential of migration among the study participants suggests however that an image about migrants as actors of development has become common as well. Important to the local production of such a public perception in Malawi may be the social experiences of return of health workers, as well as discourses and activities of transnational social actors, such as professional communities of overseas health workers (e.g. diaspora initiatives of physicians and nurses in the UK and Scotland mentioned in Lwanda 2007; Grigulis 2010) and transnational religious groups (e.g. the mentioned Seventh Day Adventist "Operation Reach Back").

The social appreciation reserved for those, who made it abroad stands in contrast with public expectation towards domestic nurses to serve in Malawi, where the common public opinion on migrating nurses has become more controversial in view of the severing crisis of human resources for health. Shifting from accepting towards disapproving attitudes (ibid.), it mirrors arguments of the political discourse. As mentioned, several students had been directly confronted with their parents' patriotic objections against migration (see p. 123). Considering that a socially disapproved migration project is associated with negative effects on social status, this national discourse presents a general threat to the students' future outlook: the accusation of abandoning one's country loosens the contract of symbolic and formalized belonging to the national community, which bears access to an institutionalized form of collective solidarity and social capital (Faist 1998) the students build upon when designing their future life plans.

Dealing with this challenge, the individual nurses struggle to position their personal migration projects as socially compatible exceptions against the background of adverse general public opinions. This reflects in a controversial ethic discussion in the group of participants: while some nurses reject any moral responsibility beyond family solidarity, most see themselves in the duty to compensate to the Malawian government or health system. Others again locate the responsibility of compensation and support with the recruiting country (see Table 9, next page).

On the one hand, most students equate personal and public concerns describing and defending an inherent necessity to migrate: they present themselves as victims of structural constraints, particularly regarding working conditions, access to further training and limited income. On the other hand, the students alleviate the conflict between their personal migration prospects and public expectations to stay by designing temporary migration projects under an umbrella of social viability.

Whereas freedom of choice and a right to free movement are commonly advanced against political restrictions on nurse migration (e.g. WS 4), measures securing that this migration should be temporary are an acceptable compromise to some students:

“As for me, I personally think that there should be programmes to determine that they should GO outside and COME back. Just do their studies and then come back. Because if you look at the nurses section, if the nurses go, that means there will be shortages, there will be more and more shortages of nurses. [...] Not just going forever and work, not coming back - which is not good. (WS 3, P21F: 21)

*Table 9. Students' Answers to: 'What would you be ready to contribute to Malawi if working abroad?'*

| |
|---|
| "If I were abroad, I would like to contribute a certain amount to help the country improve working conditions for those remaining and to train more health workers in the country." |
| "The country I am working should help my country improve working conditions." |
| "The tax of the health worker in another country should be going to the country where this individual is coming from. This should be exactly what would have been deducted in my country." |
| "10% of my salary should be sent to my home country for improving health facilities." |
| "If I were outside the country, I would prefer to lobby for my country so that the working environments should be improved hence some nurses may choose to remain here, if the working environment has improved." |
| "...advocate for Malawi to organizations abroad to assist the Ministry of Health, to change the working areas and make them conducive for nurses to work in." |
| "I can support the government in improving the hospital environment so that nurses stay back in their country." |

Long-term migration is repetitively blamed as the actual problem of nurse migration and overwhelmingly rejected on the level of the personal life plan and, generally speaking, the students affirm conformity to values of national, social and familial solidarity. Adhering to the public reservations against migration of nurses, many participants express awareness of the country's need of their services and empathy for the public anger about the losses migration of Malawian overseas nurses allegedly causes to their country.

"Researcher: […] when you are thinking about migration is it rather a decision you want to make for life, to stay there? (Several students giggling 'no!').

Participant 8F: Just to make money and come back. We can also contribute to the development of this country like building a hospital for Malawians who get old, or a psychiatric (hospital), since in Malawi we don't have that." (WS 1, P8F: 11)

"[...] if we want to add value, then we MUST get good education and then come back, develop our country. So it's still good that we go abroad, we come back, develop our country - we should be proud of our country. So we should still develop it." (WS 3, P16F: 21)

Beyond such general arguments, students discussing this issue mostly outline future plans that observe and integrate the socially common expectation that nurses would be obliged to care for their "own" people, give back their services in exchange for the education they received and contribute to the country's development. The more specific personal projects to promote development in Malawi concern and often combine material and immaterial contributions like making a change in a specific field of nursing or delivering good quality care to the poor and needy. Especially for many female students, the imagination of a successful return is connected with ideas of making charitable social investments into the local health system, e.g. building hospitals or wards with specific facilities. In some cases, charitable investments are connected with the openly expressed wish to become a socially appreciated person whose name people know, which points to the presumed relevance of such contributions for earning a high social status in Malawi.

By means of such argumentations, the students promote their temporary migration-to-study scheme as *win-win* opportunity, inscribing migration into the national project of development and building social legitimacy and admiration for their plans while protecting the expected symbolic capital of migration from public dispute. Approaching their attitudes as acquisitions of social discourses, references to the international *brain gain* discourse become obvious (see p. 10): The students defend that skilled return and investment in Malawi, remittances as well as advocacy could generate considerable social benefits for their country (WS 4; WS 5), as would returnees' transfer of skills to students and colleagues and the application of advanced and specialist skills in the Malawian health service. Whereas the students' reasoning focuses on the positive impact of migration upon return, it also considers remittances, short-term charity stays in Malawi or advocacy for the home country while abroad as beneficial results of migration. Such ideas make reference to the *migration-development mantra* (see p. 11) of *brain gain* through temporary migration and repeat elements of the newer international discourse focusing the development effects of transnational diaspora activities.

Thus, students' *brain gain* references appear in this light as personal acquisition of a convenient international discourse on migration that justifies their personal plans, establishing a second moral fundament for their ambitions to migrate, next to the universal professional ethos of nursing. Rather than as mere gesture of national and familial attachment, the personal contribution to development in Malawi may accordingly be understood as a biographical strategy to pursue a socially accepted personal status transition. The contribution to be made may then be approached as a material manifestation of the symbolic capital of migration, applied to strengthen the social capital of communal as well as familial bonds in order to pave the way for a good life back home after the envisaged return. Similarly, Herold (2008) finds that the remittances of Ghanaian migrants in Germany serve essentially to build social capital and prestige in the home society, gaining particular importance due to migrants' persistent wishes to return. The group of migrants he studied however perceive communal investments as less effective than familial ones in building the necessary social capital for a return.

The students' migration-for-development discourse highlights beyond this their broader ideas of social change as members of the

Malawian elite. As observed by Dannecker (2009), migrants' ideas and experiences of migration are often connected with diverse ideas about *development(s)*, which may encourage deep changes in the social imagination of development and modernity, depending on the power of its stakeholders. A deeper discussion of the young nurses' visions of development has not been in the focus of this study and would require looking into the specific Malawian creation of modernity and development within the modern capitalist global context (Watts 1991), which goes beyond this analysis. Nonetheless, the insights from this study suggest several dimensions of the young nurses' ideas about development.

A status-securing material approach to development *back home* is associated with socially recognized investments in the family and society: already mentioned visions to build special hospitals or services fall into this realm. Several students also resort to a discourse of national development when presenting plans to start income-generating investments or businesses in Malawi (e.g. agricultural investments and rental houses or trucks). Only in a few cases those investments are put forward however as a way to generate the freedom to nurse *"from the heart*" (WS4, P25F: 15), while they appear mostly as strategy of male nurses to forego the necessity to work in the nursing field, or as a financial security for their family-related and self-development projects.

Underlying this material dimension of development, the students general biographic approach to migration and development relates to a wishful thinking about migration as the access to the developed *Western* world, and the subsequent projection of development into the individual life plan and self (Raghuram 2009; McNeill-Walsh 2004). The young nurses' images about the destination UK absorb the master-narratives of development rooted in the colonial discourse about modernity and the superiority of the *West*. These often persist in the self-presentations of development actors: e.g. promotional literature of DFID is found to contribute to a discourse of development that allows the UK to *"[narrate] itself as a metropolitan nation that is civil, developed, modern"* Biccum (2005: 1006). Similarly and closer to the life of the nurses, the day-to-day experience in the capital Lilongwe displays development as a business of a wealthy and skilled *Western* elite: white foreigners are very visible throughout town, riding new white jeeps in the name of development cooperation organisations mentioned as funders or experts on banners all around.

Related to this discursive dimension of development, the students' approaches to development *back home* repeat already discussed colonial references of nursing. Their visions of migration are often intrinsically linked with the idea to become missionaries for modern medical care (e.g. P16F, p. 151), making their immaterial social contributions appear as symbols for the wish to modernize the *local* Malawian health system by means of the developed medicine of the *Western* world. The professional mission of developing the home country, bringing advanced nursing skills to Malawi, is not only consistent with the *brain gain* discourse, it also reproduces a common colonial reasoning of developing the colonies on behalf of *Western* nursing:

> "British nurses in the colonies were not simply purveyors of medical expertise assigned to teach modern *Western* methods to "the natives." [...] Modern *Western* medical care was understood by these women to represent the pinnacle of civilization, and thus its introduction into the colonies […] was a critical part of the broader 'civilizing mission'. […] The goal of initial training efforts was to mold Filipino nurses in the *Western*, American model as a means of bringing modern medical techniques and standards to the islands." (Schultheiss 2010: 154)

# V. BIOGRAPHIC MIGRATION PROJECTS AS POLICY ISSUE

This chapter reconsiders main findings in the light of their relevance for the political challenge to address Malawi's human resources for health crisis. Concluding, it draws together main findings from this study on the biographical dimensions of migration intentions among young nursing academics in Malawi.

## Policy Dimensions

One motivation for this study has been to inform and broaden the development political debate on nurse migration in Malawi from a biographical perspective. Limited insights into the current political health and migration management in Malawi, as well as the small research scope, however constrain a straight formulation of policy suggestions for politicians and their international development partners in Malawi. Though the study findings do not translate easily into concrete policy measures, they are of political relevance. In the following, I will therefore revisit them with a view to the migration potential of the young generation of nursing graduates in Malawi and areas of mayor political concern. Based on this, existing policies and political agendas, as well as potential approaches to be considered are discussed.

### *A Lost Generation?*

In view of the political challenge to address the human resources for health crisis in Malawi, the consequences of the study findings for the retention of young, highly qualified Malawian nurses are of foremost concern. A general concern of Malawian nursing leaders regarding the professional motivations of this upcoming generation is its supposed lack of motivation for the nursing profession and a strong trend to seek alternative employment and career opportunities upon graduation (Grigulis 2010).

Also most participants' history of recruitment into nursing makes it reasonable to assume that the lack of personal ownership in career decision-making might imply barriers to professional motivation and retention.

However, to the contrary, a strong, religiously underpinned attachment of women to the nursing profession and of men to the health sector has been observed in this study. It goes along with clear professional perspectives to pursue careers in these fields. The students' strong identification with their already obtained professional expertise and title was found to tie their professional life plans to the health sector, in many cases to different nursing specialities. As far as the overall Malawian health and nursing services are taken as points of reference, these motivations and conditions inherit potentials of retention within, or respectively return into the Malawian health system. Alternative occupations are only of concern as side activities. As Muula and Maseko (2006) show, such side jobs are among the less problematic common strategies of Malawian health workers to earn their living.

The young nurses' employment preferences for their first years of duty reflect the tendencies among public sector registered nurses in general (Mangham 2007): regarding the first workplace a commitment to serve in the public service was clearly visible. Only one participant mentioned an NGO as general preference, while far most graduates seek work in the public service, frequently mentioning district level hospitals as favourite workplace. This preference for the public sector is connected to expectations to find there the best local opportunities in terms of responsibilities on the job, working ambience and access to in-service education.

The supposition of Grigulis that the trend to migrate has been replaced by a new era of internal occupational concurrence between Malawi's public health sector and the increasing number of local NGOs did not emerge with clarity in the students' future plans. While some nurses did perceive the work in an NGO as a second option in case their migration prospects might fail, migration-to-study was generally evaluated as the priority option. This prioritization has been interpreted with regard to the symbolic value of migration, the students' perceptions about Master's programmes in Malawi and their global academic peer references. At the current point of the life course the young generation tends to place lower value on immediate financial securities than on academic opportunities and *global* experiences, supposedly connected with long-term economic benefits and professional status. In view of this, NGOs and IOs with their lack of promotional and training opportunities hardly appear as a feasible alternative, neither to migration nor to an employment in the public sector during the first years of service.

The analysis of female students' professional future concerns suggests that many do not so much avoid the challenging work at the bedside, but struggle with the status vulnerability implied by the unfortunate career conditions of a bedside nurse. As social status, including economic and lifestyle dimensions, revealed as fundamental motivation to seek professional career development and migration-to-study projects, this vulnerability is generally to be recognized as a major limitation for retention. Expecting however that as returnees their socioeconomic and academic status would be secured via savings, investments and a Master degree, several women nurses situate bedside care in their future life plan as an act of charity and social development, highlighting a high affinity to a return into this field after a successful migration project. Migration as a strategy to build savings and investments to be able to "*nurse from the heart*" (WS4, P25F: 15) may in this context also be understood as a commitment to nursing care that does not depend or rely on practices of stealing and taking extra-allowances from patients. At least under the (possibly presumptuous) preconditions of a very successful migration project, nursing care may accordingly become integral to the personal projects of status generation upon return, thus not necessarily being associated with a move away from bedside nursing forever. In the face of the strong career orientation of the nurses' lives so far, the potential for a long-term retention as middle cadres of Malawian hospitals has however to be regarded at least as questionable under the given working conditions.

### *Recognizing the Migration Potential*

The findings from this study highlight a persisting if not growing desire and perceived biographic necessity to migrate among the new generation of highly qualified nurses. Assessing the migration potential of the young generation of nursing graduates from a biographical perspective, a high individual migration potential has thus to be called into attention: migration enters the life plan as a core biographical step to realize fundamental life themes, entangling goals of professional progress, familial well-being and social development, empowerment as well as elite global and local membership. A biographic dependence on successful migration is tangible here. Though pressure to migrate from family members or partners might add to this migration potential, it did not reveal as an issue of students' concern so far. Contrariwise parents' requests to stay in Malawi were already recognized as a potential barrier to migration. On this basis it seems indicated to expect that young nurses leave as soon as opportunities arise and agreement with family members is reached.

Yet, taking into consideration the burden of political and economic challenges that the country is facing, and the decline in official nurse migration in recent years, it is plausible that the topic is not a priority on Malawi's political agenda. Whereas some stakeholders point to a persistent migration potential (VSO 2010), others tend to assume that nurse migration may not be an issue of major concern anymore (SoL 2010; Betty Mkwinda-Nyasulu and Chilemba 2007; NMCM 2010b). Muula's (2006b) analysis of sessions of the national parliament regarding the shortage of health workers highlighted a general political awareness of migration being an important factor in the shortage of health workers (mainly physicians however): the debate was torn between a consciousness that simply producing more health workers might not be enough and the attitude that politics would lack the capacity to address the problem. The then occurring changes in the UK migration regime and the subsequent decrease in official registrations of Malawian nurses to work abroad tend to be interpreted as an indication of a declining political importance of the international care drain. In turn, the political attention has shifted from international nurse migration towards dynamics of internal migration into the private health and the NGO sector (MoH 2010; Grigulis 2010).

Nonetheless, as detailed in Chapter I, dynamics of migration tend to remain volatile in the context of a high outmigration potential and given a global demand for nurses and widespread migrant networks (Bach 2003). The decline in nurses' registrations to migrate goes back to a policy shift in the main destination country, which is subject to frequent changes and beyond control of Malawian politics. As labour migration studies point out in general, the global interconnectedness of labour migration flows facilitates the establishment of new migration corridors via transnational communities and the redirection of migrants in the medium term towards countries with stronger pull-factors and easier entry (Crush, Williams and Peberdy 2005; Kingma 2007). Therefore, as noted by Kingma,

> "[n]urse migration is pushed, pulled and shaped by a constellation of social forces and determined by a series of choices made by a multitude of stakeholders. International mobility is a reality in a globalized world, one that will not be regulated out of existence." (Kingma 2007: 1294)

Though the UK has been the first destination for Malawian nurses, historically and throughout the last decades, it has not been the only one. Over the years, a strong health worker community has also established in the USA, where the census in the year 2000 counted as many Malawian nurses as in the UK (Clemens and Patterson 2008). In view of the current immigration regulations for overseas nurses, nursing graduates who destine the UK may be obliged to rethink their plans. Considering the important role of migration in many life plans it is however doubtable that they will immediately accept to stay back and look for alternative ways to pursue their professional goals in Malawi. Rather than abstaining from migration, the next generations of nurses might thus orient towards the USA or new destinations altogether to realize their migration-to-study projects. This trend has e.g. been found among Ugandan nursing graduates facing conditions similar to their Malawian colleagues (Nguyen et al. 2008) and is expected by some Malawian nursing leaders as well:

> "If they won't go to the UK, they will go to Australia. If they won't go to Australia, they will go to the US." (Ngoma quoted in VSO 2010: 16)

A comparison of NMCM registrations and census data (NSO 2009) suggests furthermore that unregistered migration might be happening and that a shift towards less formalized channels and patterns of nurse migration could be taking place. These changes could be associated with migrant nurses' adjustment to less favourable conditions of migration, raising concerns about migrants security and career prospects: if service in low-ranking care jobs becomes the only available chance to pursue a migration-to-study project, qualified nurses may be further inclined to accept deskilling working conditions. Such new patterns of Malawian nurse migration would likely compromise the opportunities to realize successful short-term migration projects and increase the risk of *brain waste* in the course of migration.

Census data[1] points furthermore to a tenfold increase in non-return emigration between 1998 and 2008, in particular in the context of further studies (NSO 2011). Though non-return numbers are naturally higher throughout recent years and the increase correlates with a steady population increase, such a sharp rise suggests an increasing importance of migration-to-study among the young qualified, calling for political action. Under these auspices, a neglect of the persistent migration potential bears the risk of overlooking dynamics of migration with a view to human resources for health planning. It is of concern to explore current shifts in migration patterns and start tracking migration and return rates of Malawian nurses, as both impact the country's *brain drain* or *brain gain* prospects and thus the political viability of migration.

The establishment of a common computerized registration database at the NMCM would be a first advancement in this area:

[1] Migration received attention in the 2008 census with questions regarding non-return emigrants' sex, age, destination, year of departure, type of activity abroad and remittances sent (NSO 2010).

during the time of data collection the manual registers of nurses seeking to work abroad were kept separately from the registers of nurses entering the Malawian nursing workforce. Tracking migration and return rates would therefore require a arduous cross-register analysis identifying cases of nurses who did not leave, despite registering to do so, and of nurses who returned into the Malawian nursing workforce.[2] In the middle perspective, the implementation of a continuous, standardized survey of migration data should be considered to retrace migration and return rates in different nursing cadres throughout nurses' professional careers. Also assessments of how migration and further studies abroad affect nurses' career progress and contribution to the local public health service in Malawi would be of interest. Taking into consideration that the aim of research should be to give a balanced picture of the phenomenon of nurse migration, it is disconcerting that Malawi is frequently cited as case in the international *brain drain* debate though no records or even estimations on return exist.

### *Strengthening Informed Decision-making*

The young nurses' migration discourse draws heavily upon idealized images of the conditions of life, nursing studies and practice abroad, as well as of a successful return connected to professional career and high social status.

With a view to the initially mentioned factors and dynamics encouraging and inhibiting migration of health workers (see Table 1, p. 13; p. 12-15), it becomes obvious that a considerable range of factors is not anticipated in the students' early migration plans: informed reflections about opportunities to study, visa and recruitment procedures, legal frameworks and practical challenges of working and studying abroad are largely absent. Barriers to migration seem either unknown or disregarded, information about international recruitment as scarce as awareness of the difficulties involved in return. Several students destining the UK expect to

---

[2] Officially an electronic nursing registry is in place since 2001 (Jhpiego 2001), however its implementation was still in progress during the time of data collection.

make arrangements on jobs before leaving, which may be regarded as a gauge of greenness with a view to the existing regulations for overseas nurses.

Instead of practical knowledge, a body of transnationally nurtured images and narratives about studying, nursing and living in *Western* countries fuels the young nurses' illusionary and wishful thinking about migrating in future. This *myth of migration* (see p. 91) might partly explain the gap between what could be regarded as reasonable biographic decision in the current global context of mobility restrictions (e.g. to seek employment with an NGO in Malawi in order to finance Master's studies in Blantyre), and the continued striving for migration-to-study projects. Considering de Jong's (2000) reasoning, that migration intentions initiate a process of migration decision-making that develops according to the person's awareness of problems and benefits involved in migration, it seems indicated to address the students' largely naïve approaches to the topic improving the preconditions for informed migration decisions as well as the eventual development of biographic alternatives to migration.

In order to assess whether and how a move abroad could further or challenge the personal biographic aspirations, more neutral and qualified information about actual conditions of migration, e.g. regulations regarding visa, study programmes, job opportunities, housing, saving etc., rights and frequent risks would be required. To come to informed and reasonable migration decisions and set up realistic plans considering resources, time-frames and benchmarks as well as alternatives to migration the students would seriously profit from counselling services. It should be considered, whether migration information and coaching for future graduates could be made available at KCN or how knowledge of and access to reliable sources of information can be promoted, e.g. via online mentoring.

Otherwise the lack of awareness about the challenges nurses' with migration-to-study projects will have to face might lead to a susceptibility to engage in riskier forms of migration and to confront failing migration and dwindling return perspectives.

### *Access to Postgraduate Studies*

While the actual role of a Master's degree for nurses' career opportunities on the local labour market requires further examination, the expected waiting time to access Master's programmes in Malawi gives well reason for migration, in particular considering the central biographic relevance of further education in the nurses' scripts of future life. The imbalance between the number of Bachelor graduates and the available MA study places in Malawi should thus be addressed: Improved access to postgraduate training is likely to open attractive biographic perspectives to nurses whose migratory motivations are largely focused on further studies. These students describe migration as 'just an opportunity' (not a fundamental building stone of their life planning), but share huge doubts with their colleagues on finding the aspired academic opportunities in Malawi.

The SWAp-Midterm Review (RoM et al. 2007) and the globalization strategy of UNIMA (2010) have long set the goal to establish more postgraduate programmes in Malawi but faced structural challenges implementing them, such as understaffing of lecturers and high costs per student due to the boarding system (RoM et al. 2007). In order to increase the number and attractiveness of locally available master study places it might be worth considering to reform the current system of full-time studies and boarding: distant learning and part-time MA programmes, combining work in the public sector with postgraduate education, seem to be more apt to cover the demands. According to a World Bank study (2004) modular or combined programmes would open possibilities to increase intakes in a cost-effective way while improving vacancy levels and encouraging locally relevant academic research at the same time. Taking the perspective of nursing students', such programmes could permit to cope with the financial burdens of further training more easily.

Beyond increasing the local postgraduate training capacities, it is important to face the restrictive regulations of nurse migration e.g. in the UK, as Malawi depends in many medical specialities on the opportunity to train its health personal abroad. Abating migration-to-study opportunities will thus likely have negative repercussions on the availability of adequately trained health professionals in the future. This raises the need to negotiate access to international training via bilateral agreements or student programmes and establish international alliances to foster postgraduate training in Malawi.

Both the CoM and KCN have been highly active in recent years to develop international cooperation in postgraduate studies: Tambulasi and Chasukwa (2011) describe an agreement between the CoM in Malawi and South African Universities, offering a five-year specialist training with three years of study in Malawi and two years in South Africa. As a measure to ensure the students' return, Malawian graduates are per agreement not allowed to work in South Africa upon completion of their studies, but facilitated in their return to Malawi. A series of new cooperation have been developed since, including partner universities in the UK and the College of Surgeons of East Central and Southern Africa (COSECSA) (CoM 2018). While there was no functioning Master's programme at KCN in 2010, currently the college offers a Master's in Child Health Nursing in partnership with the African Paediatric Fellowships Programme at the University of Cape Town in South Africa, a clinical Master's degree in Midwifery developed in partnership with the East Central and Southern African (ECSA) health community and higher education institutions, the University of Central Lancashire and WHO and a Masters degree in Reproductive Health, developed with Norwegian partners (UNB n.y.).

Programmes combining professional training and studies abroad with phases of working experience and a final research project to be conducted in Malawi might strengthen the local benefit from training opportunities abroad, maintaining bonds back home and fostering locally relevant academic research. As a tracer study on researchers from Developing Countries studying in Germany points out, the rate of returning students tends to be high if professional links are maintained and field stays conducted in the home country (Schraven, Eguavoen and Manske 2011). Universities in donor countries and health professionals in the diaspora could assist to support new training formats. An e-learning project between PHD students in Health careers at the University of Lubumbashi and the University Brussels indicates that diaspora members may contribute valuably to the realization of innovative international partnerships for professional and academic development (IOM 2007). Furthermore, the regional experiment of the Loma Linda University, offering an international MA programme in Public Health to African health graduates, bears an interesting concept to promote the academic qualifications of a Malawian and African nursing elite (Muula 2006c). The part-time structure of this programme is of particular interest, as it stretches studies over 4 years, but allows students to continue working in their home countries, even in remote areas, while furthering their education (ibid.).

A further aspect underlining the importance of such programmes is the need for a professional empowerment of Malawian nurses in (post)colonial academic relations. Nursing graduates' culture of migration-to-study as revealed in this study tends to reproduce colonial knowledge hierarchies, with few local academic references for their professional identification. Under these auspices it seems to be crucial to promote academic environments that empower Malawian nursing academics to decolonize their discipline on the basis of critical, emancipative and context-related teaching, locally, regionally and globally, building fundaments for a locally grounded nursing scholarship.

As argued by Lwanda regarding Malawian oversees physicians, there is a political need to address the unexploited potential of diaspora members to further this mission (Lwanda 2002 and 2007). In coherence with the suggestions of Lwanda, international donors should e.g. consider to support qualified return of Malawian nursing academics overseas in order to strengthen local ownership of the nursing scholarship, instead of sending more expatriate health workers to Malawi. At the same time, nursing academics in the diaspora should be encouraged to contribute to an emancipative research and teaching in their discipline.

***Restricting Mobility?***

Whereas nurse migration in a globalized world is acknowledged to be complex and not to be halted, the alarming human resource losses in some developing countries due to migration have encouraged fierce ethical and political debates. The recruitment practices of European, North American and Arab nations are criticised and a reconciliation of interests and costs between donor and recipient countries as well as migrating health workers is demanded (Lorenzo 2007; Muula 2005; Mills et al. 2008; Robinson 2008; Mundt 2011). The *"WHO Global Code of Practice on the International Recruitment of Health Personnel"* (WHO 2010), also GCP, has become a central reference in this global debate. Suggested by the code are firstly, the enhancement of bilateral or multilateral migration management via agreements, secondly, the reduction of push and pull factors in source respectively recipient countries and thirdly, the maximization of developing countries' gains from their health workers' migration. The first point of agreements is meant to improve the migration management so as to increase its benefits for the source and the destination country as well as the individual migrant, and to strengthen the international partnership for the improvement of the health workforce in developing source countries on the other hand.

Ethical recruitment guidelines also fall into the first realm. They should restrict active recruitment from countries with fragile health systems and shortages of health workers, stipulate transparent and fair recruitment conditions and lay down rights and obligations for admitted overseas health workers (Pagett and Padarath 2007). With effect to Malawian nurse migration, two main destination countries, the UK and South Africa, have implemented regulative guidelines for the recruitment and the workforce integration of overseas health workers from developing source countries. By contrast, the equally important USA has not adopted any political regulations and is still recruiting actively (Ngoma in VSO 2010).

South African policies integrate bilateral agreements promoting short-term study-and-work stays for SADC citizens with a ban of active recruitment, long-term working contracts and the hiring of

SADC health workers not applying within the frame of government-to-government agreements (ZAR 2002+2010). The successes of the UK recruitment codes have been challenged, as far as the actual impact of ethical guidelines on the reduction of active recruitment and the decline of the officially registered migration is concerned (Buchan and McPake 2007; Bach 2003).

While active recruitment from Malawi does not seem to be an issue of major concern and the students did not mention any knowledge about locally active agencies, they are affected by the regime of mobility restrictions accompanying the shifts towards policies curbing the individual immigration of overseas nurses. The UK Overseas Nursing Programme introduced in 2006 is e.g. complicating the situation of African nurses with migration-to-study projects as it delays access to MA programmes and the qualified labour market, causing prolonged stays, employment in low skilled care jobs and frustration of professional development prospects (Grigulis 2010). In 2015 the Tier 2 Visa Threshold for skilled professionals in general was raised (Travis 2015), further restricting overseas nurses' access to the UK labour market. Also the recent developments of EU nurses and domestic nurses quitting their service in the NHS (Campbell 2017) have not let to a revision of these politics. A demand of about 40.000 nurses is diagnosed, but so far the only international recruitment scheme is a temporary migration scheme with India and the Philippines to place 5,500 overseas nurses in the NHS service in the frame of bilateral 2-3 years 'earn-learn-return' agreements (Borland 2017). Despite the official policy guidelines stipulating equal entitlements for migrant and domestic nurses to access further training and professional career (Buchan and McPake 2007), African nurses' experiences of dequalification in the UK point to their de facto disadvantaged conditions for *brain gain* (Hardhill and MacDonald 2000; Henry 2007; Larsen 2007; O'Brien 2007).

Given these conditions, it is worrisome that Malawi is not only a victim of global *brain drain* dynamics: it also depends on international mobility to meet its training needs for the many medical and nursing specialities contributing to improve the quality of the local health services, an aspect of health worker mobility often ignored. Taking furthermore the future visions of a generation of young nurses serious that largely approaches migration as an essential biographic *rite of passage* (see p. 15), the promotion of short but successful stays abroad would be a better policy guidance than fierce restrictions of mobility. Taking at the same time into consideration that highly qualified migrants' are inclined to stay abroad (Baruch, Budhwar and Khatri 2007; Mundt 2011), opportunities for *brain circulation* are to be considered as important measures to improve *brain gain* from those who will establish their lives abroad (Lwanda 2002 and 2007).

***International Migration Agreements***

In view of the importance of international mobility among skilled health personal for Malawi as well as its health workers, a lopsided policy emphasis on retention is to be avoided. To profit from the international migration management agenda of the GCP, it will instead be important to involve actively in the development of bi- and multilateral agreements. These should establish political instruments to promote Malawian nurses' temporary migration-to-study opportunities, diaspora engagement and opportunities of skilled temporary or permanent return into the health sector. To design successful programmes, individual's rights of movement as well as biographic and career interests should be as much of concern as harvesting yields of migration for Malawi and its population.

Malawi has been addressing the lack of human resources trained, as well as several push factors in its health system with political commitment (see p. 20). The political management of the migration of nurses (as well as of other highly skilled professionals) has however received minor attention, as the Malawian Ministry of Labour has been hesitant to engage in this realm (SoL 2010). The apparent negligence extends to a number of International Organisations in Malawi who have been important actors in this field in other countries, e.g. IOM, ILO and WHO. Other technical agencies have so far only emphasized the aspect of retention, not of *brain circulation* and return (e.g. the SWAp-Initiative and the EHRP-Alliance). The policy lead for migration issues is currently with the Ministry of Home Affairs and Internal Security. An IOM Migration Report dating from 2014 expected this ministry to release a comprehensive citizenship and migration policy in late 2015 that should allow to address crosscutting issues of migration and development. The policy is however not available as of now and Malawi lacks experiences with bilateral agreements on migration and return, and with bilateral partnerships for professional development by means of migration (e.g. via short-term student visas and working permits or internships between health professionals from partnering countries). There are no migration-to-study-and-return schemes on national level.

A positive international example in this realm is the „Managed Migration“ Initiative of the Caribbean region: it has been implementing a range of policies that improved the win-win character of migration among countries in the region and leveraged severe shortages in several of them while respecting the health workers' rights to migrate (Salmon et al. 2007). Its success points to the potentials of thoughtful management rather than restriction of health workers' mobility, as well as to the benefits of regional cooperation policies (Buchan and Dovlo 2004). Other encouraging experiences come from a bilateral agreement between South Africa and the UK that opened two-way opportunities for health workers of both countries, e.g. short-term education and practice periods in the other country, while original posts were held open to facilitate return (WHO 2006).

In order to achieve the envisaged global partnership for migration and development, international cooperation agencies in Malawi need to examine with local stakeholders how different approaches could be implemented politically. Programmes and legal frameworks should be negotiated between regional and development partners as well as between source and destination countries. The contributions of development cooperation may compile financial support, research or consultancy to broaden the channels of temporary migration, return and transnational activity. A literature review by Buchan (2008) identifies a variety of different technical approaches that could strengthen source countries' benefits from health workers migration:

*Table 10. Examples of Potential Policy Interventions for Directing Health Worker Migration*

| **Level** | **Characteristics** |
|---|---|
| **Twinning** | Links developed by health care organizations in source and destination countries based on staff exchanges, staff support and flow of resources to source country |
| **Staff exchange** | Structured temporary move of staff to another organization, based on career and personal development opportunities or organizational development |
| **Educational support** | Educators and/or educational resources and/or funding in temporary move from destination to source organization |
| **Government-to-government bilateral agreement** | Agreement developed by destination country with source country to underwrite costs of training additional staff and/or to recruit staff for a fixed period, linked to training and development prior to staff returning to source country or to recruiting surplus staff in source country |
| **Country-level fast tracking of health worker immigration** | Preferential status or priority treatment given to health workers in terms of immigration requirements in order to speed up immigration process and facilitate active international recruitment |
| **Country-level recruitment code** | Introduction of a code by the destination country restricting employers in terms of which source countries can be targeted and/or length of stay of recruits; coverage, content and compliance issues all need to be clear and explicit |

Source: Buchan 2008: 20

Agreements and aid policies addressing the *brain drain* should be sensitive to the historically and colonially grounded roots and determinants of *brain drain* in Malawi in order to avoid a reproduction of harmful dependencies (Lwanda 2007). With regard to a reconciliation of interests researchers from the Philippines and different Sub-Saharan countries have discussed financial compensation from receiving countries as a further measure to balance lost training investments (Lorenzo 2007; Muula 2005; Mills et al. 2008; Robinson 2008). While this approach has not been practiced yet and has not been included into the GCP agenda, it could balance the burden of social responsibility migrating nurses currently have to carry alone, repeatedly to the disadvantage for successful migration projects. In a broader perspective, migration and integration policies in destination countries should address and strengthen the empowerment-through-migration potentials of migrants, protecting their rights in the personal and professional sphere and counteracting the viscous circle of gender, class, ethical and racist discrimination that, according to previous research, tends to affect (in particular female) nurses' emancipatory life projects as well as their professional progress (Larsen 2007; Smith and Mackintosh 2007).

### Promoting Engagement from Abroad

The third policy area suggested by the international migration policy discourse is based in the assumptions of the new *migration-development mantra* (Faist and Reisenauer 2009; see p. 11), as it addresses in particular the potential of diasporas to alleviate development constraints in their countries of origin. This positive approach to the linkages of migration and development is however less strong in the literature on African health workers' mobility than in the overall discourse on migration and development. The GCP remains relatively vague in this area: It requests equal opportunities for overseas health workers to access professional development and further education abroad and demands recipient and source countries to facilitate transnational activity, circular and return migration. Several studies have taken a clearer position, claiming the need for a paradigm shift away from the *brain drain* perspective and towards a more balanced assessment of welfare losses, gains, dangers and potentials of African health workers' migration for 'development' (Padarath et al. 2003). They suggest recipient countries to adapt visa frameworks and release barriers to the transfer of savings and social security benefits, making temporary or permanent return more viable. Source countries are encouraged to strengthen their ties to health workers overseas, empowering their diaspora communities to engage with their home countries' health institutions and setting up incentives and support schemes for temporary or permanent physical return (Haour-Knipe and Davies 2008). Lwanda (2007) insists in a strong potential for diaspora engagement of Malawian physicians overseas if viable schemes of engagement would be available.

In many countries, the recognition that large amounts of remittances flow back from migrants has let governments to increase their efforts to build stronger relations with diaspora communities in general. Yet, for Malawi formal remittance sending remains (despite substantial increases) very low according to official numbers, which could be an effect of informal money transfer methods being common. (Ndegwa 2014) Despite this, diaspora engagement has become an issue in Malawian politics, both on the ministerial level and in development cooperation. New policies and programmes seem to be underway since the establishment of a Diaspora Unit at the Ministry of Foreign Affairs and International Cooperation in 2012 (MFAIC 2013). The EU MIEUX Initiative, IOM and ICIRD are supporting the ministry's efforts in diaspora engagement with expertise since 2014 (ibid.; MIEUX 2016). In view of these developments, the findings of Muula (2006b) on Malawi's national policy discourse regarding migration of health professionals may also have shifted from the assumption of political powerlessness and an understanding of migration as *brain drain* towards the recognition of possibilities to address the diaspora potentials inherent to this migration. Desk study however suggests that the attempted steps to build diaspora linkages are taken very slowly: the process of developing a Diaspora Engagement

Policy, started in 2014, has apparently not been finalized, nor has the undertaking to hold a Homecoming Summit in 2016. For June 2018 the Malawi Embassy in the USA has invited for a first high-ranking diaspora conference and announced the meeting would be the first step in a process towards establishing a platform enhancing diaspora engagement for development in Malawi (Malawi Embassy 2018).

While these developments are likely to open opportunities of engagement to migrant health workers, none of the activities had or has its focus here. The current scale of diaspora activity among Malawian health workers overseas, their contributions to the local health system and their potential engagement remain still as unexplored as the return rates of nurses. Considering the young graduates' discourse about development and their social aspirations in Malawi, they are likely to feel attracted by opportunities to make social contributions to their home country. The concrete needs of overseas nurses willing to become involved in health issues in Malawi as well as ways to support different forms of overseas nurses' diaspora engagement should thus be clarified. Existing experiences of small initiatives like the Scotland-based diaspora initiative MIND (Malawi Initiative for National Development) and the mentioned Adventist diaspora in the USA might be helpful in this regard: both facilitate temporary work stays in Malawi (Grigulis 2010; MIND 2011; Mkwinda-Nyasulu and Chilemba 2007). Studies by international development organisations expect that the promotion of temporary return could motivate more overseas nurses to engage in Malawi and propose that the strengthening of diaspora links should become integral to the national policies addressing medical *brain drain* (Tambulasi and Chasukwa 2011; VSO 2010), which is not the case so far.

Beyond the attempts of source countries like Malawi to strengthen ties with migrant communities, destination countries like the UK and the USA could actively support *brain gain* from nurses in the diaspora: the loosening of regulations, which lead to a loss of citizenship entitlements upon leaving the country, and making arrangements to improve the transferability of social security benefits for the years of service abroad are two important issues to look into.

### *Opening Return Prospects*

The possibilities to determine based on this study the return potential of those who will find chances to migrate are very limited. Their return decisions will depend on unpredictable migration experiences and conditions and their current return plans hardly bear realistic orientations as they rely on vague images and difficultly practicable projects of migration. Furthermore, aspirations and discourses of return tend to persist even among long-term migrant nurses who postpone their return projects continuously due to various social, professional and economic constraints (VSO 2010; Herold 2008). However, potential impediments and resources for later return can be stressed.

The euphemistic collective expectations of social status transition via migration tangible in the cohort of young graduates may discourage them from an envisaged return as has been described for nurses in the UK, facing familial and social expectations regarding professional progress and income generation abroad, which they were not able to satisfy (VSO 2010; Grigulis 2010.

"You know a colleague went to the UK, and you know in the UK there is money, you wouldn't expect her to come back empty handed. You would want her to come back, for her to be better than you. They have to be different from the way they left otherwise we people who stayed in Malawi would laugh at them, why did you go to UK? What have you benefited? You left your family, how different are you?" (Female nurse quoted in Grigulis 2010: 187)

At the point when young overseas nurses will have to evaluate concretely their realistic chances after studies against the expected ones, their enthusiastic ideas about life after return are likely to hinder the homecoming, especially of those whose migration projects were less successful and whose career opportunities back home do not promise social advancement. As migration studies have documented, return intentions of highly skilled migrants in general often fail due to own, family and society's unrealistic expectations towards returnees' success and wellbeing. In particular highly skilled migrants often decide to extend their stay abroad after their studies, when evaluating opportunities in the host country against those in their country of origin (Baruch, Budhwar and Khatri 2007; Mundt 2011).

Furthermore, as suggested by Larsen et al. (2005), nurses migrating at a young age are more inclined to consider a move with the family and stay for longer periods. This trend could apply to nursing students sharing a common migration project with their couple and who are likely to carry responsibility for children abroad at the point of finishing their studies, i.e. when considering return - a return difficulty found commonly among overseas students after finishing their Master studies (Baruch, Budhwar and Khatri 2007). That migration often develops to be a project of the whole family has furthermore been suggested by findings for overseas nurses in the UK, where a majority had taken their children with them, despite differences according to nurses' origin (Buchan et al. 2006). Migrants' strong social relatedness to the society of origin while abroad may furthermore lead to the acceptance of professional and status degradation in the destination country over a longer timespan, bearing risks for successful return (Parnreiter 2000 on the theory of dual labour markets of M. J. Piore).

Ideas of national solidarity and social contributions back home are a recurrent argument for return, but are also connected with aspirations of social status. They are far from new in Malawi, as they can be traced back to the promotion of patriotism under the Banda regime and have since never kept health workers from staying abroad (Lwanda 2007). It has been argued in the literature that strong social bonds back home and optimism to generate improved personal, economic and social status in the home country may translate into a major factor of return migration, if the latter come to be realistic (Chappell and Glennie 2010; Haour-Knipe and Davies 2008). Regarding return migration of highly skilled professionals, the ability to achieve specific labour market, educational or financial goals is highly relevant in the case of short-term migration projects (Chappell and Glennie 2010). The young nurses' positive visions of future life and professional career in Malawi may thus be regarded as an important resource that, if maintained and furthered throughout the migration project, might encourage a return.

Though the rampant wishful thinking about migration in unlikely to be fulfilled, the attractiveness of return may be preserved as long as fundamental professional needs connected with the *rite of passage* of migration can be met. This would likely be the case e.g. when nurses leave for short-term stays abroad, generating specialist academic knowledge and small savings and chances of a labour market entry at an advanced level upon return. Adequate conditions for short, academically successful migration projects and fast re-entry into responsible positions of the labour market have been crucial to enhance long-term return perspectives for highly qualified nurses in other contexts (ibid.; Haour-Knipe and Davies 2008) and will likely be critical in Malawi as well. This links to the complex endeavour to strengthen professional development, tackled in the next chapter. Also provisions to supply overseas nurses with local health labour market information systematically, and the offering of employment support, saving schemes and entrepreneurial information etc. could be considered on the part of the Malawian government to assist successful and sustainable return.

Optimistic attitudes towards return distinguish the young nurses from many health workers in other African countries (Awases et al. 2004): According to findings of a cross-country WHO study, the feeling to have “no future” in the home country presents an important reason to leave in these countries (ibid.). It correlates for Zimbabwean university students with a trend to seek long-term migration (Tevera 2005). Malawi's high political stability and job security for nurses throughout the past decade may explain in parts the greater optimism among Malawians, drawing attention to the possible effects of the country's increasing political and socioeconomic fragility since 2011. According to Grigulis (2010) and a personal conversation with an older overseas nurse's sister, political factors had already been an important aspect of long-term nurse migration from Malawi during the Banda regime.

At the same time, it has to be taken into account that nurses returning to serve in bedside nursing in Malawi, will likely face difficulties to cope with the harsh conditions of the fragile health system they are facing. NONM spokesperson Dorothy Ngoma illustrates this, stating that

> "[w]hen health workers do come back from working overseas, most do not go to the bedside. Our low level system with its inadequate resources and lack of equipment makes meeting the needs of intensive care very hard work. It's traumatic psychologically when there is nothing you can do for people dying of things that they shouldn't. [...] They can come back physically, but not to where they were. If they do, they will not last because they can't cope. You can't blame them. It is an impossible task – we are asking them to do something none of us can." (Ngoma quoted in VSO 2010: 10)

### *Making Nursing in Malawi Attractive*

The second policy approach of the GCP demands to address health system related push and pull factors of health workers' migration from developing countries. In low income developing countries, international development cooperation is requested to assist source countries with their human resources for health training, retention, management and planning. Conjoint initiative and investment should improve the working and payment conditions of health workers and the quality of health care, therewith containing the disease burden and the number of health workers required. Educational and financial incentives, regulatory measures as well as social and professional support are proposed by the GCP to address the global and local misdistribution of health workers. (WHO 2010)

Many of these recommendations have been tackled within the agenda of Malawi's Emergency Human Resource Programme, a joint effort of the Malawian government and its international development partners: the programme was able to increase training capacities for degree and diploma cadres, introduced locum incentives, salary top-ups as well as bonding schemes, and improved human resource planning capacities (see p. 20). It was successful to relieve the immediate shortage and sustaining its measures would likely improve the future availability of health workers in the Malawian public health system. Also the practice of channelling applicants of UNIMA into the nursing career was stopped before 2010 already, as KCN saw the shortfalls and had sufficient first-choice applications (Grigulis 2010). In order to improve retention rates, it might furthermore be indicated to bring more experienced nurses than young academic best-performers into the career, redistributing training capacities from the BSc Nursing and Midwifery towards the post-basic bachelor programme in nursing. The increase of training capacities remains however a first step only. Issues of professional development and continued education of nurses, which have been identified as a particular important for retention in Malawi (MSH 2009; Tambulasi and Chasukwa 2011), go beyond the emergency programme and need to be addressed specifically.

Former studies have suggested that professional development might be gaining weight within the professional motivation of future generations of Malawian nurses (Grigulis, Prost and Osrin 2009). The study findings strengthen this suggestion indirectly as they point to the particular importance of academic habitus and individual career prospects in young nurses' biographic future plans. A career-ambitious professional identity is of high importance to their self and social identities as well as status goals, connected with visions about membership to the Malawian academic elite and exceptional contributions to the improvement the health care for Malawians. Most students accept the necessity to collect working experience at the bedside within the two obligatory years of duty following their studies. But they commonly mention reservations about a long-term occupation in Malawi's public health sector, making reference to different challenges to professional development there, including a lack of encouraging and appreciative supervision, access to further training, and entitlements to participate in managerial and care-related decision-making. Furthermore, many students expect that their degree of qualification would not be valued appropriately and that their whish to be awarded responsible functions might be frustrated. Last but not least, the subordination of nurses to similarly trained clinician cadres emerges as a concern in this area. Several students pointed strongly to a frustration about the political representation of their professional development interests by the NMCM and the MoH. Progressing in nursing was seldom translating into a vision about being a matron, but rather into aiming at a specialization in (mostly) paediatric nursing and reproductive health or in public health, with envisaged occupational areas in preventive health at community level, research and teaching, health policy making, health management or awareness and advocacy work.

Connected with such wishes to work in the areas of illness prevention, awareness raising and community work, areas largely limited to health related NGOs and IOs in Malawi, an attractiveness of employment at alternative health providers becomes visible upon the envisaged return: Nursing graduates might seek jobs with NGOs to pursue their thematic interests; reciprocally, their thematic foci on these areas might implicitly reflect a career orientation towards job prospects in the better paying NGO environment. Dorothy Ngoma, cited above, sees the harsh conditions of hospital care as most important reason for returnees fleeing into NGO and private sector jobs, raising the need to work towards serious improvements of bedside nurses' working conditions if retention is to be achieved (VSO 2010).

Given the negative expectations of recent nursing graduates towards a career in the public health service, the reform process of the human resources for health management as well as the career development regulations of the NMCM should consider emphasizing the particular career concerns of young, academically trained nurses. As high vacancy rates in the health sector are present on all levels of the occupational hierarchy, the health managerial and political career motivations of highly qualified nurses bear a valuable potential to fill higher posts. Training more young ambitious students in the Bachelor of Nursing programme without being able to open academic and occupational career perspectives to them upon graduation is otherwise likely to result in low retention rates and little gains from the higher training efforts and costs. The study findings underline the previous suggestions of Tambulasi and Chasukwa (2011) that clear and attractive occupational career paths in nursing will be strongly appreciated by highly trained cadres more generally. While the concern about professional development is outstanding in the students' professional life projects, it is not limited to them. On the contrary, the implementation of clear job positions and career paths as well as professional development schemes in order to improve retention has also been suggested from research on other cadres (Manafa et al. 2009; Muula and Maseko 2006).

A nursing cadre hierarchy and career paths are officially in place (see Annex Table 2), the reality of promotion has however been outlined as an area of frustration for highly qualified nurses due to delays, arbitrariness and restrictions to enter upper health management functions (MoH 2010+2011a; RoM et al. 2007; see p. 33-34; Table 7, p. 70). Career paths should integrate performance-oriented opportunities for a fast career development, early participation in management decisions and a fair competition between nurses and clinicians in the middle and higher health management. The MoH could also evoke the introduction of a young professionals programme to improve the public sector's reputation in terms of straight career opportunities, and to strengthen the early recruitment and retention of qualified and motivated junior staff to the Ministry and build trainees' capacities to perform in responsible functions. Also small measures might help to address the disadvantages of young professionals in the hospital environment, such as reserving a seat for a representative of young professionals in the hospital management board, strengthening the learning against the control aspect of supervision and considering young professionals in the selection for in-service trainings. Development agents may contribute to such efforts financially and with consultancy. Securing access to professional development and further education, and valuing academic training within the hospital system are likely to improve the retention of highly qualified nurses in a more effective way than bonding schemes. The latter had not been reinforced with legal consequence by 2010, but the establishment of a tracking system was envisaged for 2016 (MoH 2011b).

From a gender perspective, the subordinated, feminized position of nursing in the health system leads to nurses' frustrations about their decision-accomplishing rather then decision-making tasks, their lower rank than similarly qualified male-dominated health worker cadres and their moderate remuneration. Reforms that improve the professional status of nursing in relation to clinical cadres would thus be to the benefit of both female and male nurses. More controversial are reforms which open promotional opportunities, attractive management posts and straight career paths, as they may generate disadvantages for women nurses in a patriarchal system, where male job candidates tend to be preferred over females for managerial and leadership positions (Evans 2004; Tracey and Nicholl 2007). In Britain, the new 'Salmon' management system introduced into the NHS with the objective of "*bringing in a more business-like ethos, with improved efficiency*" (Evans 2004: 326) is seen as one of such reforms, by which

> "management positions were 'made ripe for male capture' (p. 197 [Salmon report]). By emphasizing the need for promotion based on merit and proven administrative ability, Dingwall (1972) points out that men nurses, despite poor formal educational qualifications, were positioned to take advantage of leadership jobs." (Ibid.)

These developments allowed the relatively low share of men in nursing in the UK to outnumber women in leadership and management positions by far, implying an intrusion of patriarchal hierarchies within the traditionally female-dominated profession (Evans 1997 and 2004). Also the generally female-dominated Malawian nursing service has experienced a run of male nurses on leadership and decision-making positions with male graduates foregoing bedside-nursing and entering immediately into management positions or NGO placements (Grigulis 2010; Tambulasi and Chasukwa 2011). Grigulis (2010) reveals that nursing officials' scepticism regarding male nurses' avoidance of the bedside has let to a reduction of male intakes in higher cadres, especially on degree level: KCN intake rates of men to the Bachelor of Nursing programme dropped from 16 out of 19 intakes in 2004 to approximately one third in 2010 (KCN 2010). Beyond a mere politics of quotas, the promotion of empowering experiences of supervision and recognition abroad and in Malawi could be a rewarding path to a more positive professional identity and commitment among Malawian men in nursing, as the case of a male nursing student with internship experience in Finland suggests (P15M, see p. 98).

At the current point in their biographies, female nursing graduates may be able to defend their career ambitions in competition with male colleagues as their career plans mirror the straightness described by Tracey and Nicholl:

> "Younger women now are more likely to plan their careers and career pathways and to structure their personal lives around these plans. They establish careers before marriage and/or having children. Younger women also choose work environments where gender-based prejudices are less pronounced, and as part of their career plan, they choose partners who will be more likely to assist rather than block their plans (Scase and Goffee 1990)" (Tracey and Nicholl 2007: 678).

In view of the gendered embedding of women nurses in family responsibilities, they may however have to adapt their plans and resort to circular career paths as soon as obligations and priorities in other life projects need to be coped with, which might then put them in a misfortunate position towards male colleagues. Beyond questions of women nurses' professional stake, the analysis has highlighted that different aspirations of empowerment are woven into their future and migration projects. Regarding a future and return perspective of women nurses in Malawi, the findings are of relevance in the context of approaches to enhance women's empowerment.

In view of the social situation of women in Malawi (see p. 22-24; Table 5, p. 61), it is tangible that female nursing graduates count with an exceptional position: as the percentage of women with higher education is low, women nurses represent an important proportion of Malawi's academically educated women and their social background, professional commitment and self-consciousness are for the most part supportive of an engagement in responsible positions and leadership. Considering the gender gaps in leadership, it appears to be a social imperative to promote the career ambitions of these young women: as of 2013, women officers only occupied 23% of decision-making positions in the Civil Service and women are also highly underrepresented in non-governmental leadership structures as well as political representation (GoM 2013; Kayuni 2017). If female nursing graduates' are to be retained to fill vacant posts at the middle and upper level of the public health care service, their biographic priority on professional career challenges health management politics to open career paths and professional development opportunities for their cadre, and to renegotiate the position of nursing as a feminized profession within the hierarchy of health professions. Beyond nursing, there is a need to encourage the higher education of women in other academic fields, loosening the focus on and supporting girls' performance in science subjects. The original career choices of the female nursing students presented a broad spectrum of professional preferences but they were channelled into nursing by UNIMA's focus on MSCE grades in science subjects, impeding girls' admission in many programmes. Grigulis (2010) describes how the criteria for admission into different UNIMA subjects are clustered along the MSCE performance in different subjects, with science grades being an effective hurdle for women to enter technical careers, though lower entrance conditions have been implemented for girls in science subjects (Gomile-Chidyaonga 2003).

## Conclusions

The main objective of this study has been to broaden the analytical approach towards the migration of Malawian nurses from a biographic perspective. In view of this, the study has explored the biographic anchorage of migration intentions in different life projects as well as the overall future perspectives of young nursing graduates in Malawi. It strengthens the argument of Findlay et al. (2012) that migration intentions of students should be treated in the frame of their overall life plans as it has pointed out how migration intentions build into students' life concepts, future plans and aspirations, often assigning an essential biographic function to migration.

Analysing how young nursing students respectively graduates approach migration as part of their wider biographic projects, the chapters of this book have demonstrated the crucial importance of migration to the realization of their ambitious future life plans: the role of migration has been traced in seven different areas of the young nurses' biographic outlook. This allowed exploring a complexity of linkages between their life scripts, self- and social identities, their professional, familial and personal situation and the shapes of their different intentions and biographical ideas on migration. The analysis shows that individuals' migration-to-study intentions are situated at the interface of their family-, partnership- and self-related perspectives of future, in between religious guidance, gender concepts, academic habitus and (post)colonial images.

Four overarching observations can be highlighted: Firstly, although the assessed biographic projects reflect only the students' current aspirations and plans, they make reference to migration as a substantial and encompassing *life theme* (Keddi 2008), entangling values and *biographical horizons* that establish an enduring orientation for the life plan (see p. 45). The young nurses tend to arrange their biographic plans in a sequence of migration and a subsequent stage of successful return. Their personal migration projects thus correspond to a biographic future concept that is directed towards a good life in the Malawian, not the destination country's society and labour market. At the same time, their future life becomes situated within different global, transnational as well as local settings.

Secondly, migration functions within the young nurses' life plans as a biographic strategy to acquire resources, which are expected to be inaccessible in Malawi, but important to reach an elite social and economic status in the local society. These resources comprise the *cultural capital* of academic education, the *social capital* of membership in an international community of the skilled and privileged, the *economic capital* of personal savings and higher income as well as the *symbolic capital* of migration as a manifestation of privilege and success. As the young nurses attribute particular biographic importance to the development of their *cultural capital*, their migration projects can be classified in the first place as migration-to-study projects, associated with symbolic connotations of development, empowerment and success.

Thirdly, the students' intention to gather these resources by means of migration is fuelled by a transfigured (post)colonial perspective on the opportunities of development accessible in the modernized *West*. Their affinity to migrate ties up with a transnational habitus historically cultivated among Malawian nursing academics. It is this context and social image that anchors the participation in a global community of the privileged as a biographic *rite of passage* (see p. 15) pursued to obtain personal development and elite social status in Malawi.

Fourthly, the different migration projects are grounded in the conflictive constellation of the young nurses' individualistic life scripts and elite self-identities, and a social context of gender roles, family expectations and local employment conditions limiting their ambitions of self-determination, career and social mobility. Under these circumstances the students' approach migration as a socially compliant strategy of self-empowerment and self-development. This implies a generational tendency towards individually shaped migration projects, in which the urgency of a move abroad is evaluated mainly in terms of the individual life agenda. Socio-economic expectations of the family, necessities of partners and children as well as caring responsibilities towards family members in the case of women nurses shape the students' ideas of their future, but constitute challenges and interferences to these individual migration projects. Building harmony between personal migration intentions and constraining social expectations is the dominant biographic strategy encountered in the examined life plans. In most cases, this harmony is associated with the design of mutually beneficial temporary migration projects, though single women with highly individualistic life scripts and the wish to overcome gender-related forms of biographic heteronomy in Malawi escape this picture and lean towards visions of long-term migration.

In summary, it can be concluded from the analysis that the young graduates’ migration intentions concentrate on the generation of elite biographic perspectives in Malawi, the participation in a global community and self-empowerment. While social concerns and family contexts influence the envisaged migration projects, those arise in the first place from an individual biographic agenda to reach a social status that is determined by norms in the global and local social spaces the young academic nurses consider as their frame of reference. The individuals' biographic planning mobilizes a mental infrastructure of migration that is built upon social associations between migration and privilege, reproduced traditions of academic migration in the nursing profession and an appropriation of the social identity of a progressive and globalized social elite.

Revisiting these findings in an analytic meta-perspective, an interplay of different individual and social conditions, local and global influences as well as historical and current transnational dynamics reveals as the substance of the students' biographic approaches to migration. Table 11 (next page) names the main factors of relevance to the shapes of the nurses' migration projects on different levels of influence, ranging from the individual to the global.

These insights embed the technical knowledge about push and pull factors of international nurse migration explored by previous research in highlighting the biographic relevance of specific social, professional and individual motivations to migrate among graduated nurses. The biographic perspective contextualizes economic push and pull factors of nurse migration, highlighting the linkages between economic wellbeing and the graduates' distinctive positions in family and society, clashing with the economic conditions of nurses in Malawi. Relating the study findings to the typology of migrant nurses by Kingma (see p. 15-16) the study thus contributes an integral perspective on migration intentions, showing that different types merge and interact in the biographical migration projects of young nursing graduates.

*Table 11. Malawian Nursing Students' Biographic Approach to Migration*

| | |
|---|---|
| **Individual Preconditions** | Embodied cultural and social capitals facilitating migration<br>Degree of social embedding and determination vs. degree of individualization and appropriation of personal entitlements<br>personal and social status aspirations<br>Strategic acquisition of global and local resources<br>Information/awareness of local and global chances/challenges |
| **Local Embedding** | Family and social expectation of reciprocity and status<br>Social and gender norms of the public life-course<br>Local discourse on migration and development<br>Professional status of nursing and accessibility of status progress |
| **(Post)colonial Heritage** | Idealised images about nursing in Britain Colonial linkages and traditions of migration Professional status of nursing and accessibility of status progress |
| **Trans-nationalism** | Cultures of nurse migration and academic migration<br>Religious transnationalism |
| **Globalization** | Global nursing and academic markets<br>Global mobility culture of the highly-skilled<br>Images about globally available resources and lifestyles |

In contrast to findings by Grigulis (2010) on biographies of former generations of overseas nurses from Malawi, aspects of empowerment and individualization through migration show in the young nurses' life plans with equal importance as aspects of social responsibility and reciprocal family contract. The migration intentions are reasoned within an individual life course perception that recognizes personal entitlement to make life and lifestyle choices, as well as to draw on globally available resources to progress individually while protecting social bonds.

As this study has been focusing individual biographic perceptions, it did not allow exploring the influence of family norms and roles on the young nurses' migration intentions into depth, e.g. the aspect of shifting influences between core and extended families. While it hints at an individualization trend in migration intentions and presumed decisions, this finding needs to be further scrutinized by research addressing itself to the (gendered) family dynamics of young nursing graduates' migration decision-making, as well as by investigations into shifting biographic orientations towards migration throughout different life stages.

The findings are consistent with Grigulis' (2010) push and pull model of nurse migration, as far as the importance of recognition, better allocation and promotion policies and further training opportunities are concerned. They put flesh on the observations of Grigulis, Prost and Osrin (2009) about a more career-oriented new generation of Malawian nurses. And they raise assumptions on the specificity of nursing graduates' migration intentions due to their academic environment, their individualistic orientation, professional ambition, elite status and global reference points - aspects to be treated as specific to the students' current life stage, family status and awareness of conditions of the local and the global labour market.

However, as has been highlighted for the field of lifestyle migration in particular (see p. 130-32), the mental geographies of migration and privilege among the highly skilled are globalizing to a certain extend, creating within African countries like Malawi reflections of migratory phenomena attributed to the developed world. Beyond concrete challenges related to conditions of employment, postgraduate education and independent lifestyles in Malawi, the study points particularly to the subtle influence of self-identities and social imaginations that devaluate local and appreciate global conditions of professional and personal development. Associations between migration, progress and status are exposed on the individual and social level as a symbolic capital of migration and a vital element of nurses' perpetuating *culture of migration*. Further comparative studies on the North-North and South-North migration of students may be useful to deepen the understanding of common dynamics and differences in this respect. A comparison of the study results with biographical perceptions of students in other nursing cadres in Malawi would be required to evaluate whether the identified dynamics are specific to graduates or whether they extend to other groups of nurses.

The discussion of political consequences deriving from the study results has pointed to the need to gain comprehensive statistical knowledge about *brain drain* and *brain gain* potentials from nurses' migration. To take an informed political position towards this migration, some core technical questions for further research will be: did and do nurses who are registered to go abroad really leave, improve their capacities abroad and build relevant professional knowledge to contribute to health service provision in Malawi? Which occupational functions do returning nurses take and do they apply qualifications gained abroad? Which kind of support would be required to facilitate informed decisions for migration, temporary or permanent return as well as to strengthen diaspora engagement? Astonishingly, despite the still vibrant development political discourses of *brain drain* and *brain gain* and the attention Malawi received for several years as a case of international migration of nurses, the country has hardly received any interest by scholars or International Organisations in this respect. I thus hope that the findings from this study will still be useful and inspiring to further research and that some of the policy considerations may find their way into political debates on the migration of health workers from Malawi and beyond.

Last but not least, the entangling of a *myth of migration* with nurses' idealized ideas of return and development, indicates a need to study how the current *brain gain* discourse inscribes into an idealised (post)colonial narrative of migration. An important question for policy research will then be how migrant Malawian nurses can empower themselves professionally to contribute to an emancipation of their discipline from this (post)colonial heritage.

## *Literature References*

Aboderin, Isabella. 2007. "Contexts, motives and experiences of Nigerian overseas nurses: understanding links to globalization." *Journal of Clinical Nursing*. 16(12): 2237–2245.

Akl, Elie A., Nancy Maroun, Stella Major, Claude Afif, Bechara Chahoud, Jacques Choucair, Mazen Sakr, and Holger J. Schünemann. 2007. "Why are you draining your brain? Factors underlying decisions of graduating Lebanese medical students to migrate." *Social Science & Medicine.* 64(6): 1278–1284.

Alonso-Garbayo, Álvaro, and Jill Maben. 2009. "Internationally recruited nurses from India and the Philippines in the United Kongdom: the decision to emigrate." *Human Resources for Health.* 7: 37.

Arango, Joaquin. 2000. "Explaining migration: a critical review." *International Social Science Journal.* 52 (165): 283-296.

Awases, Magda, Akpa R. Gbary, Jennifer Nyoni, and Rufaru Chatora. 2004. *Migration of Health Professionals in six Countries: A synthesis report.* South Africa: WHO Regional office for Africa.

Bach, Steven. 2003. "International migration of health workers: Labour and social issues." *ILO Working Paper.* Geneva: International Labour Organisation.

Baldassar, Loretta, Cora Vellekoop Baldock, and Raelene Wilding. 2007. *Families Caring Across Borders: Migration, Ageing and Transnacional Caregiving.* New York: Palgrave MacMillan.

Ball, Rochelle E. 2004. "Divergent development, racialised rights: globalised labour markets and the trade of nurses—The case of the Philippines." Women's Studies International Forum 27: 119–133.

Baruch, Yehuda, Pawan S. Budhwar, and Naresh Khatri. 2007. "Brain drain: Inclination to stay abroad after studies." *Journal of World Business.* 42(1): 99–112.

Bastia, Tanja. 2011. "Migration as protest? Negotiating gender, class, and ethnicity in urban Bolivia." *Migration as protest? Negotiating gender, class, and ethnicity in urban Bolivia.* 43(7): 1514-1529.

Bauman, Zygmunt. 2000. "Social Issues of Law and Order." *British Journal of Criminology.* 40(2): 205-221.

Bauman, Zygmunt. 1998. *Globalization: the Human Consequences.* Oxford: Polity.

Benson, Michaela and Karen O'Reilly. 2009. "Migration and the search for a better way of life: a critical exploration of lifestyle migration." *The Sociological Review*. 57(4): 608-625.

Bhabha, Homi K. 1996. "Cultures in Between." *In Questions of Cultural Identity.,* ed. Stuart Hall and Paul Du Gay. London: Sage, pp. 53-60.

Bhargava, Alok, Frédéric Docquier, Yasser Moullan. 2011. "Modeling the effect of physician emigration on human development." *Economics and Human Biology.* 9(2): 172-183.

Biccum, April R. 2005. "Development and the 'New' Imperialism: a reinvention of colonial discourse in DFID promotional literature." *Third World Quarterly.* 26(6): 1005-1020.

Bloor, Michael. 2001. *Focus Groups in Social Research.* London: Sage.

Bonnett, Alastair. 2003. "From White to Western: 'Racial Decline' and the Idea of the West in Britain, 1890–1930." *Journal of Historical Sociology* 16(3): 320-348.

Borland, Sophie. 2017. "NHS hires 5,500 'rolling' nurses from abroad: Staff will work in the UK for up to three years before returning home." *Daily Mail Online*. Last modified November 29 2017, http://www.dailymail.co.uk/news/article-5127091/NHS-hires-5-500-rolling-nurses-abroad.html.

Boswell, Christina. 2008. "Combining Economics and Sociology in Migration Theory." *Journal of Ethnic and Migration Studies.* 34(4): 549-566.

Bourdieu, Pierre. 1998. *Practical reason.* Stanford: Stanford University Press.

Bourdieu, Pierre. 1986. "The forms of capital." In *Handbook of Theory and Research for the Sociology of Education.,* ed. John G. Richardson. New York: Greenwood, pp. 241-258.

Boyd, Monica, and Elizabeth Grieco. 2003. "Women and Migration: Incorporating Gender into International Migration Theory." *Migration Policy Institute*. Last modified March 01 2003, http://www.migrationinformation.org/Feature/print.cfm?ID=106.

Buchan, James. 2008. "How can the migration of health service professionals be managed so as to reduce any negative effects on supply?" *WHO Policy Brief to the European Observatory on Health Systems and Policies.* Copenhagen: WHO.

Buchan, James, and Barbara McPake. 2007. *The Impact of the Department of Health, England, Code of Practice on International Recruitment.* Edinburgh: Queen Margaret University.

Buchan, James, Renu Jobanputra, Pippa Gough, and Ruth Hutt. 2006. "Internationally recruited nurses in London: a survey of career paths and plans." *Human Resources for Health.* 4(14).

Buchan, James, and Delanyo Dovlo. 2004. *International Recruitment of Health Workers to the UK: A Report for DFID.* London: DFID Health Systems Resource Centre.

Buchmann, Marlis. 1998. *The Script of Life in Modern Society. Entry into Adulthood in a changing World.* Chicago/ London: The University of Chicago.

Butler, Judith. 2004. *Undoing Gender.* New York/ Abington: Routledge.

Campbell, Denis. 2017. "European nurses and midwives leaving UK in droves since Brexit vote." *The Guardian.* Last modified November 2 2017, https://www.theguardian.com/society/2017/nov/02/european-nurses-midwives-leaving-uk-nhs-brexit-vote.

Chappell, Laura and Alex Glennie. 2010. "Show Me the Money (and Opportunity): Why Skilled People Leave Home - and Why They Sometimes Return." Migration Policy Institute. Last modified April 2010, http://www.migrationinformation.org/Feature/display.cfm?id=779.

Charmaz, Kathy C.. 2006. *Constructing Grounded Theory*. A Practical Guide Through Qualitative Analysis. London: Sage.

Chimombo, Joseph P. G., Mike Chibwanna, Chris Dzimadzi, Esme Kadzamira, Esther Kunkwenzu, Demis Kunje, and Dorothy Namphota. 2000. "Classroom, School and Home Factors that Negatively Affect Girls' Education in Malawi." *Report to UNICEF.* Centre for Educational Research and Training. Last modified 2000 [Draft], http://www.unicef.org/spanish/evaldatabase/files/MLW_2000_005.pdf.

Chimwaza, Wanangwa, Effie Chipeta, Andrew Ngwira, Francis Kamwendo, Frank Taulo, Susan Bradley, and Eilish McAuliffe. 2014.

"What makes staff consider leaving the health service in Malawi?" *Human Resources for Health*. 12(17).

Clemens, Michael A., and Gunilla Pattersson. 2008. "New data on African health professionals abroad." *Human Resources for Health.* 6(1).

CoM (Malawi College of Medicine). 2018. *Postgraduate Programmes.* Accessed February 1 2018, https://www.medcol.mw/postgraduate-programmes/.

Crush, Jonathan, Vincent Williams, and Sally Peberdy. 2005. "Migration in Southern Africa." *Paper prepared for the Policy Analysis and Research Programme of the GCIM (Global Commission on International Migration).* Accessed February 20 2018, http://www.iom.int/jahia/webdav/site/myjahiasite/shared/shared/mainsite/policy_and_research/gcim/rs/RS7.pdf.

CSR (Centre for Social Research, University of Malawi). 2007. *Malawi Health Sector Employee Census.* Lilongwe: Ministry of Health.

Dannecker, Petra. 2009. "Migrant Visions of Development: A Gendered Approach." *Population, Space and Place.* 15(2): 119-132.

Dannecker, Petra. 2005. "Transnational Migration and the Transformation of Gender Relations: The Case of Bangladeshi Labour Migrants." *Current Sociology.* 53(4): 655–674.

Dannecker, Petra. 2003. "The Constructing of the Myth of Migration: Labour Migration from Bangladesh to Malaysia." *Working Paper.* No. 345. Bielefeld: Sociology of Development Research Center.

Davison, Jean. 1993. "School Attainment and Gender Attitudes of Kenyan and Malawian Parents towards educating girls." *International Journal of Educational Development.* 13(4): 331-338.

De Jong, Gordon F. 2000. "Expectations, gender, and norms in migration decision-making." *Population Studies.* 54(3): 307-319.

DESA (Department of Economic and Social Affairs). 2004. World Survey on the Role of Women in Development. Women and International Migration. New York: United Nations.

DFID (UK Department for International Development). 2015. "Annual Review 2014/15 of the Malawi Health Sector Support Programme.

Summary Sheet." *UK AID Development Tracker.* Accessed August 20 2017, https://devtracker.dfid.gov.uk/projects/GB-1-202214/documents.

DFID (UK Department for International Development). 2014. "Annual Review 2013/14 of the Malawi Health Sector Support Programme. Summary Sheet." *UK AID Development Tracker*. Accessed August 20 2017, https://devtracker.dfid.gov.uk/projects/GB-1-202214/documents.

DFID (UK Department for International Development). 2010. "Evaluation of Malawi's Emergency Human Resources Plan." *EHRP Final Report.* Cambridge: Management Science for Health.

Docquier, Frédéric, and Hillel Rapoport. 2011. "Globalization, Brain Drain and Development." *Discussion Paper.* No. 5590. Bonn: Institute for the Study of Labour (IZA).

Docquier, Frédéric, B. Lindsay Lowell, and Abdeslam Marfouk. 2008. "A Gendered Assessment of the Brain Drain." *Policy Research Working Paper.* No. 4613. The World Bank Development Research Group.

DoH UK (UK Department of Health). 2004. *Code of Practice for the International Recruitment of Healthcare Professionals*. London: DoH.

Dovlo, Delanyo. 2003. *The Brain Drain and Retention of Health Professionals in Africa.* Case study prepared for a Regional Training Conference on 'Improving Tertiary Education in Sub- Saharan Africa: Things That Work!' Accra, September 23-25. http://www.worldbank.org/afr/teia/conf_0903/dela_dovlo.pdf

Durevall, Dick, and Richard Mussa. 2010. *Employment Diagnostic Analysis on Malawi prepared to the Government of Malawi.* Geneva: International Labour Organisation.

Englund, Harri. 2004. "Cosmopolitanism and the Devil." *Ethnos.* 69(3): 293–316.

Englund, Harri. 2003. "Christian Independency and Global Membership: Pentecostal Extraversions in Malawi." *Journal of Religion in Africa.* 33(1): 83-111.

Evans, Joan. 2004. "Men nurses: a historical and feminist perspective." *Journal of Advanced Nursing.* 47(3): 321–328.

Evans, Joan. 1997. "Men in nursing: issues of gender segregation and hidden advantage." *Journal of Advanced Nursing.* 26(2): 226–231.

Faist, Thomas. 1998. "Transnational social spaces out of international migration: evolution, significance and future prospects." *European Journal of Sociology.* 39(2): 213-247.

Faist, Thomas, and Eveline Reisenauer. 2009. "Introduction: Migration(s) and Development(s): Transformation of Paradigms, Organisations, and Gender Orders." *Sociologus.* 59(1): 1-16.

Featherstone, Mike. 1987. "Lifestyle and Consumer Culture." *Theory Culture & Society.* 4(1): 55- 70.

Fern, Edward F. 2001. *Advanced focus group research.* Thousand Oaks, California: Sage.

Findlay, Allan M., Russell King, Fiona M. Smith, Alistair Geddes, and Ronald Skeldon. 2012. "World class? An investigation of globalisation, difference and international student mobility." *Transactions of the Institute of British Geographers.* 37(1): 118–131.

Forster, Peter G. 1997. "Religion and the State in Tanzania and Malawi." *Journal of Asian and African Studies.* 32(3-4): 163-184.

Giddens, Anthony. 1991. *Modernity and self-identity. Self and society in the late modern age.* Cambridge: Polity Press.

Giddens, Anthony. 1995. "Affluence, Poverty and the Idea of a Post-Scarcity Society." *UNRISD Discussion Paper.* No. 63. United Nations Research Institute for Social Development.

Glaser, Barney G., and Anselm L. Strauss. 2005. *Grounded Theory: Strategien qualitativer Forschung.* Bern: Huber.

GoM (Government of Malawi), and UNDP (UN Development Programme). 2002. "The Impact of HIV/AIDS on Human Resources in the Malawi Public Sector." *Report.* http://www.hrhresourcecenter.org/node/1403.

GoM (Government of Malawi), 2013. *Joint Sector Strategic Plan of the Gender, Children, Youth and Sports Sector Working Group 2013-2017.* Accessed February 5 2018, http://www.gender.gov.mw/index.php/downloads/resources/ministry-of-gender-children-and-social-welfare/9-the-joint-sector-strategic-plan-2013-2017/file.

Gomile-Chidyaonga, Flossie A. 2003. *Encouraging greater enrolments of women in science and technology: the Malawi Polytechnic experience.* Case study prepared for a Regional Training Conference on 'Improving Tertiary Education in Sub-Saharan Africa: Things That Work!' Accra, September 23-25. Accessed February 20 2018, http://siteresources.worldbank.org/INTAFRREGTOPTEIA/Resources/flossie_gomile.pdf.

Gottfredson, Linda S. 2005. "Applying Gottfredson's Theory of Circumscription and Compromise in Career Guidance and Counseling." In *Career Development and Counseling: Putting Theory and Research to Work.,* ed. Steven D. Brown and Robert W. Lent. Hoboken, New Jersey: John Wiley and Sons, pp. 71-100.

Gottfredson, Linda S. 1981. "Circumscription and compromise: A developmental theory of occupational aspirations." *Journal of Counseling Psychology.* 28(6): 545–579.

Grigulis, Astrida I. 2010. *Lives of Malawian nurses: Stories behind the statistics*. Thesis for the degree of Doctor of Philosophy. London: University College.

Grigulis, Astrida I., Audrey Prost, and David Osrin. 2009. "The lives of Malawian nurses: the stories behind the statistics." *Transactions of the Royal Society of Tropical Medicine and Hygiene.* 103(12): 1195-1196.

Grovogui, Siba N. 2010. "The *Global South*: A Metaphor, Not an Etymology." *Global Studies Review.* 6(3).

Günther, Marga. 2008. "Ausgestaltung und Aushandlung – Die Analyse der Forschungssituation als Erkenntnisinstrument." *Soziale Probleme.* 19(1): 53-71.

Hallam, Julia. 2000. *Nursing the image: media, culture, and professional identity*. London: Routledge.

Haour-Knipe, Mary and Anita Davies. 2008. *Return Migration of Nurses.* Geneva, Philadelphia: International Centre on Nurse Migration.

Hardhill, Irene, and Sandra MacDonald. 2000. "Skilled International Migration: The Experience of Nurses in the UK." *Regional Studies.* 34(7): 681-692.

Henry, Leroi. 2007. "Institutionalized disadvantage: older Ghanaian nurses' and midwives' reflections on career progression and stagnation in the NHS." *Journal of Clinical Nursing.* 16(12): 2196–2203.

Herold, Sebastian. 2008. „When you are tired you have to go home! Rücküberweisungen und Zukunftsvisionen von Ghanaern in Deutschland." *Hausarbeit zur Erlangung des Akademischen Grades eines Magister Artium.* Mainz: Johannes Gutenberg Universität.

Hunt, Stephen. 2002. "`Neither Here nor There': The Construction of Identities and Boundary Maintenance of West African Pentecostals." *Sociology.* 36(1): 147–169.

IOM (International Organisation of Migration). 2007. *Health worker migration in South and Southern Africa: Literature review*. Pretoria: IOM.

IPU (Inter-Parliamentary Union). 2015. *Malawi National Assembly. General Information*. Accessed August 20 2017, http://www.ipu.org/parline-e/reports/2195.htm.

Izuhara, Misa, and Hiroshi Shibata. 2002. "Breaking the chain of the generational contract? Japanese migration and old-age care in Britain." In *The transnational family: New European frontiers and global networks.*, ed. Deborah Bryceson and Ulla Vuorela. Oxford: Berg, pp. 155-169.

Jamison, Dean T. and Marlaine E. Lockheed. 1985. "Participation in Schooling: Deferminants and Learning Outcomes in Nepal." *Education and Training Series Report.* No. EDT9. World Bank and Education and Training Department.

Jhpiego. 2002. *Strengthening capacity to monitor training and licensure of nurses and midwifes: the Malawi experience*. Information Sheet. Last modified November 2002, http://pdf.usaid.gov/pdf_docs/pnacr729.pdf.

Joint Learning Initiative. 2004. *Human Resources for Health. Overcoming the crisis.* Cambridge, Massachusetts: Harvard College.

Kadzamira, Esme C. 2003. *Where has all the education gone in Malawi?* Brighton: Institute of Development Studies, University of Sussex.

Kamwendo, Martha. 2010. „Constructions of Malawian boys and girls on gender and achievement." *Gender and Education.* 22(4): 431-445.

Kasente, Deborah. 2006. *Gender and social security reform in Africa.* Paper to the SADC Social Security Specialists Conference `Gender and Social Security in the SADC-Region'. www.fesnam.org/pdf/2006/events/No10_PaperKasente.pdf.

Kayuni, Happy M. 2017. In Malawi, gender gaps persist despite popular support for equal opportunity. Dispatches No.152. Accessed February 9 2018, http://afrobarometer.org/publications/ad152-malawi-gender-gaps-persist-despite-popular-support-equal-opportunity.

KCN (Kamuzu College of Nursing). 2010. *Data sheet on KCN intakes between 2006 and 2010*. Requested in December 2010. [Unpublished].

Keddi, Barbara 2008. "Junge Frauen: Vom doppelten Lebensentwurf zum biografischen Projekt." In *Handbuch Frauen- Und Geschlechterforschung,* ed. Ruth Becker and Beate Kortendiek. Wiesbaden: VS Verlag für Sozialwissenschaften, pp. 428-433.

Keddi, Barbara 2003. *Projekt Liebe. Lebensthemen und biographisches Handeln junger Frauen in Paarbeziehungen*. Opladen: Leske und Budrich.

Kingma, Mireille. 2007. "Nurses on the Move: A Global Overview." *Health Services Research.* 42(3): 1281-1298.

Kingma, Mireille. 2006. *Nurses on the Move: Migration and the Global Health Care Economy.* Ithaca, New York: University Press.

Larsen, John A. 2007. "Embodiment of discrimination and overseas nurses' career progression." *Journal of Clinical Nursing.* 16(12): 2187–2195.

Larsen, John A., Helen T. Allan, Karen Bryan, and Pam Smith. 2005. "Overseas nurses' motivations for working in the UK: globalization and life politics." *Work Employment Society.* 19(2): 349-368.

Lewin, Keith M., and Yusuf Sayed. 2005. *Non-Government Secondary Schooling in Sub-Saharan Africa. Exploring the Evidence in South Africa and Malawi*. Sussex: Centre for International Education, University of Sussex.

Levitt, Peggy. 2003. "You Know, Abraham Was Really the First Immigrant": Religion and Transnational Migration." *International Migration Review.* 37(3): 847-873.

Levitt, Peggy. 1996. “Social Remittances: A Conceptual Tool for Understanding Migration and Development.” *Working Paper Series.* No. 96.04. Cambridge, Massachusetts: Harvard University, Center for Population and Development Studies.

Likupe, Gloria. 2006. “Experiences of African nurses in the UK National Health Service: a literature review.” *Journal of Clinical Nursing.* 15(10): 1213-1220.

Lorenzo, Fely M. E., Jaime Galvez-Tan, Kriselle Icamina, and Lara Javier 2007. “Nurse Migration from a Source Country Perspective: Philippine Country Case Study.” *Health Services Research.* 42(3): 1406-1418.

Luethi, Barbara. 2005. “Transnationale Migration - Eine vielversprechende Perspektive?” *H-Soz-u- Kult*. Last modified April 13 2005, http://hsozkult.geschichte.hu-berlin.de/forum.

Lwanda, John. 2002. “Doctoring the Brain Drain: Medical Case of Malawi.” *African Issues.* 30(1): 47-51.

Lwanda, John. 2007. “Scotland, Malawi and Medicine: Livingstone’s Legacy, I Presume? An Historical Perspective.” *Scottish Medical Journal.* 52(3): 36-44.

Mackintosh, Carolyn. 1997. “A historical study of men in nursing.” *Journal of Advanced Nursing.* 26(2): 232– 236.

Mahowe, Mylen. 2005. “Characteristics of Respondents and Women's Status.” In *Malawi National Demographic and Health Survey 2004,* 25-53. Zomba: National Statistical Office and Calverton, Maryland: ORC Macro.

Malawi Embassy. 2018. *Malawi Diaspora Conference 2018.* Accessed February 2 2018, http://www.malawiembassy-dc.org/MWDiasporaUSA.

Maluwa-Banda, Dixie. 2004. “Gender sensitive educational Policy and Practice: The Case of Malawi.” *Prospects.* 34(1): 71-84.

Mangham, Lindsay. 2007. “Addressing the Human Resource Crisis in Malawi’s Health Sector: Employment preferences of public sector registered nurses.” *Economic and Statistical Analysis Unit (ESAU) Working Paper.* No. 18. London: Overseas Development Institute.

Manafa, Ogenna, Eilish McAuliffe, Fresier Maseko, Cameron Bowie, Malcolm MacLachlan, and Charles Normand. 2009. "Retention of health workers in Malawi: perspectives of health workers and district management." *Human Resources for Health.* 7(65).

Massey, Douglas S., Joaquin Arango, Graeme Hugo, Ali Kouaouci, Adela Pellegrino and J. Edward Taylor. 1993. „Theories of International Migration: A Review and Appraisal." *Population and Development Review.* 19(3): 431-466.

Massey, Douglas S., Joaquin Arango, Graeme Hugo, Ali Kouaouci, Adela Pellegrino, and J. Edward Taylor. 1998. *Worlds in Motion. Understanding International Migration at the End of the Millennium.* Oxford: Clarendon.

McCoy, David, Barbara McPake, and Victor Mwapasa. 2008. „The double burden of human resource and HIV crises: a case study of Malawi." *Human Resources for Health,* 6(16).

Mchakulu, Japhet E. J. 2007. "Youth Participation in Radio Listening Clubs in Malawi." *Journal of Southern African Studies.* 33(2): 251-265.

McNeil-Walsh, Colleen. 2004. "Widening the Discourse. A Case for the Use of Post-Colonial Theory in the Analysis of South African Nurse Migration to Britain." *Feminist Review.* 77: 120-124.

MFAIC (Ministry of Foreign Affairs and International Cooperation). 2013. *Diaspora Services. Current Activities.* Accessed February 2 2018, http://www.foreignaffairs.gov.mw/index.php/diaspora-services/current-activities.

MIEUX Initiative (Migration EU Expertise). 2016. *Malawi Diaspora Affairs*. Accessed February 3 2018, https://www.mieux-initiative.eu/en/actions/165-malawi-diaspora-affairs.

Mills, Edward J., William A. Schabas, Jimmy Volmink, Roderick Walker, Nathan Ford, Elly Katabira, Aranka Anema, Michel Joffres, Pedro Cahn, and Julio Montaner. 2008. "Should active recruitment of health workers from sub-Saharan Africa be viewed as a crime?" *The Lancet.* 371: 685-688.

MIND (Malawian Initiative for National Development). 2011. *MIND Pilot Report 2009-2010.* Accessed October 11 2011, http://www.mind-uk.org//scripts/download.php?key=3A8473FF&file=mind-pilot-report.pdf&format=pdf.

Mkwinda-Nyasulu, Betty, and Winnie Chilemba. 2007. "The extend and impact of skills migration on Malawi's scientific and technological sector: the nursing profession." *Research presented to the Capacity Building Workshop 'Diaspora Knowledge Networks' as a source for Human Capital*, 28 May, 2007. Malawi: Kamuzu College of Nursing and Bunda College in collaboration with the University of Dundee. [Unpublished].

MoH (Ministry of Health Malawi) 2015. *2014/15 Annual Review Report for the Health Sector*. Lilongwe: Ministry of Health.

MoH (Ministry of Health Malawi). 2011a. *Nurse/Midwife Training Operational Plan. Field Assessments, Analysis and Scale-up Plans for Nurse Training Institutions*. Lilongwe: Ministry of Health.

MoH (Ministry of Health Malawi) 2011b. *Health Sector Strategic Plan 2011-2016. Moving Towards Equity and Quality.* Lilongwe: Ministry of Health.

MoH (Ministry of Health Malawi). 2010. *Definition of Nursing Cadres. Grade K-E*. Department of Nursing Service. [Unpublished].

Moreno-Fontes Chammartin. 2008. "Migration, Gender Equality and Development." *Overview Paper of the International Conference on gender, migration and development: seizing opportunities, upholding rights*. September 25-26. Manila, Philippines: International Labour Office. Accessed February 20 2018, http://www.ilo.org/manila/whatwedo/eventsandmeetings/WCMS_124726/lang--en/index.htm.

MSH (Management Science for Health). 2009. *Report on a Study on Performance Appraisal Systems in the Health Sector in Malawi*. Lilongwe: GTZ Health [Draft].

Mundt, Hans W. 2011. "Brain-Drain aus Afrika – Emigrieren die besten Köpfe in den Norden?" In *Herausforderung Afrika. Gesellschaft und Raum im Wandel,* ed. Johannes M. Nebe, Baden-Baden: Nomos, pp. 193-208.

Muula, Adamson S. 2005. "Is There any Solution to the "Brain Drain" of Health Professionals and Knowledge from Africa?" *Croatian Medical Journey.* 46(1): 21-29.

Muula, Adamson S. 2006a. "Nationality and country of training of medical doctors in Malawi." *African Health Sciences.* 6(2): 118-119.

Muula Adamson S. 2006b. "Shortage of health workers in the Malawian public health services system: how do parliamentarians perceive the problem?" *African Journal of Health Sciences.* 13(1): 124-130.

Muula, Adamson S. 2006c. "My Africa. Training Public Health Professionals in Africa: Loma Linda University Approach." *Croatian Medical Journal.* 47(3): 512-514.

Muula, Adamson S., and Fresier Maseko. 2006. "How are health professionals earning their living in Malawi?" *BioMed Central Health Services Research.* 6: 97.

Muula, Adamson S., Yohane Nyasulu, and Gladys Msiska. 2004a. "Gender distribution of students and staff at the University of Malawi College of Medicine, 1991-2003." *South African Medical Journal.* 94(8): 636-637.

Muula, Adamson S., Yohane Nyasulu, and Gladys Msiska. 2004b. "Gender distribution of teaching staff and students at the Kamuzu College of Nursing, Malawi 1979-2001." *African Journal of Health Sciences.* 11(1-2): 74-76.

Muula, Adamson S., Ben Panulo, and Fresier C. Maseko. 2006. "The financial losses from the migration of nurses from Malawi." *BioMed Central Nursing.* 5: 9.

Ndegwa, David. 2014. *Migration in Malawi. A Country Profile.* Geneva: IOM. http://publications.iom.int/system/files/pdf/mp_malawi.pdf.

Nguyen, Lisa, Steven Ropers, Esther Nderitu, Anneke Zuyderduin, Sam Luboga, and Amy Hagopian. 2008. "Intent to migrate among nursing students in Uganda: Measures of the brain drain in the next generation of health professionals." *Human Resources for Health.* 6: 5.

Ngwira, Naomi, Garton Kamchedzera, and Linda Semu. 2003. "Malawi: Strategic Country Gender Assessment (SCGA)." *Main Report. Vol. 1, presented to the World Bank and UNDP.* http://siteresources.worldbank.org/EXTAFRREGTOPGENDER/Resources/MalawiSCGA.pdf.

Nieswand, Boris. 2011. "Der Migrations-Entwicklungs-Nexus in Afrika. Diskurswandel und Diasporaformation ." In *Potenziale der Migration zwischen Afrika und Deutschland,* ed. Tatjana Baraulina, Axel Kreienbrink and Andrea Riester. Nürnberg and Eschborn: Bundesamt für Migration und Flüchtlinge and Deutsche Gesellschaft für Internationale Zusammenarbeit, pp. 400-425.

NMCM (Nursing and Midwifery Council of Malawi). 2010a. *Manual review of the registration books between 2004-2010.* [Unpublished].

NMCM (Nursing and Midwifery Council of Malawi). 2010b. *Personal conversation with the NMCM registrar.* [Unpublished].

NONM (National Organisation of Nurses and Midwives) and Cordaid. 2010. "Soon there will be no angels on earth." *Billboard Advertisement.* [digital image] Retrieved March 3 2018 from https://nanm.tumblr.com/

NSO (National Statistical Office of Malawi). 2009. "Population Characteristics". *2008 Population and Housing Census Results.* Statistical tables. Accessed Mai 23 2011, http://www.nso.malawi.net/images/stories/data_on_line/demography/census_2008/Main%20Report /Statistical%20tables/Population%20Characteristics.xls

NSO (National Statistical Office Malawi). 2010. *Migration Report of the 2003 Malawi Population and Housing Census.* Accessed Mai 23 2011, http://www.nso.malawi.net/images/stories/data_on_line/demography/census_2008/Main%20Report /ThematicReports/Migration%20Report.pdf.

NSO (National Statistical Office), and ICF Macro. 2011. *Malawi Demographic and Health Survey 2010.* Zomba, Malawi: NSO, and Calverton, Maryland, USA: ICF Macro. http://www.nso.malawi.net/index.php?option=com_content&view=article&id=175:the-2010- malawi-demographic-and-health-survey-2010-mdhs&catid=8&Itemid=46.

O'Brien, Terri. 2007. "Overseas nurses in the National Health Service: a process of deskilling." *Journal of Clinical Nursing.* 16(12): 2229-2236.

OECD (Organization for Economic Cooperation and Development). 2008. "The Looming Crisis In the Health Workforce. How can OECD countries respond?" *OECD Health Policy Studies.* OECD Publishing.

Omaswa, Francis. 2009. "Health Worker Migration: Perspectives from an African Health Worker." In *Realizing the Right to Health,* ed. Andrew Clapham et al.. Zürich: Rüffer & Rub, pp. 436-445.

Orozco, Manuel, Lindsay Lowell, and Johanna Schneider. 2006. "Gender-Specific Determinants of Remittances: Differences in Structure and Motivation." *Report to the World Bank Group, Gender and Development Group, PREM.* Last modified March 10 2012 [Draft], http://siteresources.worldbank.org/INTGENDER/Resources/Session2Orozcoetal.pdf.

Padarath, Ashnie, Charlotte Chamberlain, David McCoy, Antoinette Ntuli, Mike Rowson, and Rene Loewenson. 2003. "Health Personnel in Southern Africa: Confronting maldistribution and brain drain." *EQUINET Discussion Paper.* No. 3.

Pagett, Catherine, and Ashnie Padarath. 2007. "A review of codes and protocols for the migration of health workers." *EQUINET Discussion Paper.* No. 50.

Palamuleni, Martin E. 2011. "Socioeconomic determinants of age at marriage in Malawi." *International Journal of Sociology and Anthropology.* 3(7): 224-235.

Parnreiter, Christof. 2000. "Theorien und Forschungsansätze zu Migration." In *Internationale Migration: die globale Herausforderung des 21. Jahrhunderts?,* ed. Karl Husa, Christof Parnreiter, and Irene Stacher. Frankfurt: Brandes&Apsel, 25-52..

Penton, James M. [1997] 1999. *Apocalypse delayed: the story of Jehovah's witnesses.* Reprint ed., Toronto, Buffalo and London: University of Toronto Press.

Pessar. 1999. "Engendering migration studies: the case of new immigrants in the United States." *American Behavioral Scientist.* 42(4): 577-600.

Piper, Nicola. 2008. "International Migration and Gendered Axes of Stratification. Introduction." In *New perspectives of gender and migration: livelihood, rights and entitlements,* ed. Nicola Piper. Geneva: UNRISD Research in Gender and Development and New York: Routledge, pp. 1-34.

Pond Bob, and Barbara McPake. 2006. "The health migration crisis: the role of four Organisation for Economic Cooperation and Development countries. " *The Lancet* 367: 1448–1455.

Raghuram, Parvati. 2009. "Caring about `brain drain´ migration in a postcolonial world." *Geoforum.* 40(1): 25-33.

Robinson, Mary, and Peggy Clark. 2008. "Forging solutions to health worker migration." *The Lancet.* 371(9613): 691-693.

Robb, Nadia, Lisa Dunkley, Petra Boynton, and Trisha Greenhalgh. 2007. "Looking for a better future: Identity construction in socio-economically deprived 16-year olds considering a career in medicine." *Social Science & Medicine.* 65(4): 738–754.

RoM (Republic of Malawi), Ministry of Health, Malawi Health SWAp Donor Group, and GTZ. 2007. *Human Resources/Capacity Development within the Health Sector. Needs Assessment Study.* Final Report.

Ross Sara J., Daniel Polsky, and Julie Sochalski. 2005. "Nursing shortages and international nurse migration." *International Nursing Review.* 52(4): 253–62.

Salmon, Marla E., Jean Yan, Hermi Hewitt, and Victoria Guisinger. 2007. "Managed Migration: The Caribbean Approach to Addressing Nursing Services Capacity." *Health Services Research.* 42(3 Part II): 1354-1372.

Schraven, Benjamin, Irit Eguavoen, and Günther Manske. 2011. "Capacity Development durch Bildungsmigration: Ergebnisse einer Befragung von afrikanischen Entwicklungsforschern." In *Potenziale der Migration zwischen Afrika und Deutschland.,* ed. Tatjana Baraulina, Axel Kreienbrink and Andrea Riester. Nürnberg and Eschborn: Bundesamt für Migration und Flüchtlinge and Deutsche Gesellschaft für Internationale Zusammenarbeit, pp. 293-313.

Schultheiss, Katrin. 2010. "Imperial Nursing: Cross-Cultural Challenges for Women in the Health Professions: A Historical Perspective." *Policy, Politics, & Nursing Practice.* 11(2): 151-157.

Schultz, Ulrike. 2014. „'Über Daten nachdenken': Grounded Theory Studien in der entwicklungssoziologischen Forschung." In *Qualitative Methoden in der Entwicklungsforschung.* ed. Petra Dannecker and Birgit Englert. Wien, Mandelbaum, pp. 75-93.

Skeldon, Ronald. 2005. "Globalization, Skilled Migration and Poverty Alleviation: Brain Drains in Context." *Working Paper.* No. T15.

Brighton, UK: Development Research Centre on Migration, Globalization and Poverty, University of Sussex.

Smith, Pam, and Maureen Mackintosh. 2007. "Profession, market and class: nurse migration and the remaking of division and disadvantage." *Journal of Clinical Nursing.* 16(12): 2213–2220.

SoL (Secretary of Labour Malawi). 2010. Letter in response to a request for a personal interview. Ref-No. 1/2/55. [Written communication].

Strauss, Anselm L., and Juliet M. Corbin. 1990a. *Basics of qualitative research: Grounded theory procedures and techniques.* Newbury Park: Sage.

Strauss, Anselm L., and Juliet M. Corbin. 1990b. "Grounded Theory Research: Procedures, Canons and Evaluative Criteria." *Zeitschrift für Soziologie.* 19(6): 418-427.

Sweetman, Paul. 2003. "Twenty-first century dis-ease? Habitual reflexivity or the reflexive habitus." *The Sociological Review.* 51(4): 528-549.

Tambulasi, Richard I.C. and Chasukwa, Michael. 2011. *Study on Measures against Brain Drain in the Health Sector in Malawi.* Submitted to the Malawi German Health Programme. [Unpublished].

Tambulasi, Richard I.C. and Chasukwa, Michael. 2015. "Holding the brains back in: an assessment of measures against brain drain in the Malawian health sector." *Africa Review.* 7(2): 104-120.

Tevera, Daniel S. 2005. "Early Departures: The Emigration Potential of Zimbabwean Students." *Migration Policy Series.* No. 39. Cape Town: Southern African Migration Project (SAMP).

Tracey, Catherine, and Honor Nicholl. 2007. "The multifaceted influence of gender in career progress in nursing." *Journal of Nursing Management.* 15(7): 677-682.

Travis, Alan. 2015. "Nurses to be among first affected by plan to cut skilled migration." *The Guardian.* Last modified June 10 2015, https://www.theguardian.com/uk-news/2015/jun/10/nurses-to-be-first-group-affected-by-plan-to-reduce-skilled-migration.

Tung, Rosalie L. 2008. "Brain circulation, diaspora, and international competitiveness." *European Management Journal.* 26(5): 298-304.

UK NMC (Nursing and Midwifery Council of the United Kingdom). 2003. *Statistical Analysis of the Register 1 April 2002 to 31 March 2003*. Accessed December 10 2010, http://www.nmc-uk.org/Documents/Statistical%20analysis%20of%20the%20register/NMC%20Statistical%20analysis%20of%20the%20register%202002%202003.pdf.

UK NMC (Nursing and Midwifery Council of the United Kingdom). 2004. *Statistical Analysis of the Register 1 April 2003 to 31 March 2004*. Accessed December 10 2010, http://www.nmc-uk.org/Documents/Statistical%20analysis%20of%20the%20register/NMC%20Statistical%20analysis%20of%20the%20register%202003%202004.pdf.

UK NMC (Nursing and Midwifery Council of the United Kingdom). 2005. *Statistical Analysis of the Register 1 April 2004 to 31 March 2005*. Accessed December 10 2010, http://www.nmc-uk.org/Documents/Statistical%20analysis%20of%20the%20register/NMC%20Statistical%20analysis%20of%20the%20register%202004%202005.pdf.

UK NMC (Nursing and Midwifery Council of the United Kingdom). *Statistical Analysis of the Register 1 April 2005 to 31 March 2006*. Accessed December 10 2010, http://www.nmc-uk.org/Documents/Statistical%20analysis%20of%20the%20register/NMC%20Statistical%20analysis%20of%20the%20register%202005%202006.pdf.

UK NMC (Nursing and Midwifery Council of the United Kingdom). 2007. *Statistical Analysis of the Register 1 April 2006 to 31 March 2007.* Accessed December 10 2010, http://www.nmc-uk.org/Documents/Statistical%20analysis%20of%20the%20register/NMC%20Statistical%20analysis%20of%20the%20register%202006%202007.pdf.

UK NMC (Nursing and Midwifery Council of the United Kingdom). 2008. *Statistical Analysis of the Register 1 April 2007 to 31 March 2008*. Accessed December 10 2010, http://www.nmc-uk.org/Documents/Statistical%20analysis%20of%20the%20register/NMC%20Statistical%20analysis%20of%20the%20register%202007%202008.pdf.

UK NMC (Nursing and Midwifery Council of the United Kingdom). 2011. *Data requests from the UK NMC Registrar: 11/2010 and 08/2011*. [Email conversation].

UN-DESA (Department of Economic and Social Affairs). 2005. *2004 World Survey on the Role of Women in Development. Women and International Migration*. New York: United Nations.

UNB (University of New Brunswick). No Year. *Kamuzu College of Nursing.* Accessed February 1 2018, http://www.unb.ca/exchange/outgoing/qeii/commonwealth_community/partners/academic_partners/kcn.html.

UNFPA (United Nations Population Fund). 2006. "A Passage to Hope. Women and International Migration." *UNFPA State of World Population 2006.* New York: UNFPA.

UNIMA (University of Malawi). 2010. *UNIMA Strategy for addressing Implications of Globalization in Higher Education.* Last modified November 29 2010 [Draft]. http://www.maastrichtuniversity.nl/web/file?uuid=f4ce3153-347e-4364-a8d1- 7ab689a3dbd9&owner=d174c69d-dc91-4ffc-9d0c-57eb26120861.

Van Dijk, Rijk A. 2002. "Religion, reciprocity and restructuring family responsibility in the Ghanaian Pentecostal diaspora." In *The transnational family: New European frontiers and global networks,* ed. D. Bryceson and U. Vuorela, Oxford: Berg, pp. 173-196.

Van Blerk, Lorraine, and Nicola Ansell. 2006. "Imagining migration: Placing children's understanding of 'moving house' in Malawi and Lesotho." *Geoforum.* 37(2): 256-272.

Vásquez, Manuel A. 2009. "The Global Portability of Pneumatic Christianity: Comparing African and Latin American Pentecostalisms." *African Studies.* 68(2): 273-286.

Vinokur, Anni (2006): "Brain migration revisited", *Globalisation, Societies and Education*. 4(1): 7-24.

VSO (Volunteer Services International). 2010. "Brain Gain. Making Health Worker Migration work for rich and poor countries." *VSO briefing: the perspective from Africa*. London: VSO UK.

Watts, Michael J. 1991. "Mapping Meaning. Denoting Difference, Imagining Identity: Dialectical Images and Postmodern Geographies." *Geografiska Annaler. Series B, Human Geography.* 73(1): 7-16.

Weyl, Ulrich. 1980. *Labour migration in Malawi as a barrier to development*. Osnabrück: University of Osnabrück.

WHO (World Health Organisation). 2006. *The World Health Report 2006: Working together for health.* Geneva: WHO.

WHO (World Health Organisation). 2010. "WHO Global Code of Practice on the International Recruitment of Health Personnel." *Resolution*: WHA63.16. http://apps.who.int/gb/ebwha/pdf_files/WHA63/A63_R16-en.pdf.

WHO (World Health Organisation) 2014. "Global Health Expenditure Database." Accessed August 09 2017, http://apps.who.int/nha/database/ViewData/Indicators/en.

World Bank. 2004. "Cost, Financing and School Effectiveness of Education in Malawi. A future of limited choices and endless opportunities." *Africa Region Human Development Working Paper Series.* World Bank Development Research Group.

World Bank 2010. "The Educational System in Malawi." *World Bank Working Paper.* No. 182. Washington D.C.: The Bank for International Reconstruction and Development/ The World Bank.

ZAR (Republic of South Africa). 2002. "Policy on recruitment, employment and support of foreign health professionals in the Republic of South Africa." *ZAR Department of Health*. Accessed August 10 2011, http://www.rudasa.org.za/download/dohpolicy02.doc.

ZAR (Republic of South Africa). 2010. "Employment of Foreign Health Professionals in the South African Health Sector as approved by the National Health Council." *ZAR Department of Health*. Accessed August 10 2011, http://www.doh.gov.za/docs/policy/2010/fwm_policy.pdf.

Zlotnik, Hania. 2003. "The Global Dimensions of Female Migration." *Migration Policy Institute*. Last modified September 23 2011, http://www.migrationinformation.org/Feature/display.cfm?id=109%20#.

## *Picture References*

Dibelius, Olivia. Berlin.

# Data References

| Abbreviation | Document cited | Date | Duration |
|---|---|---|---|
| Interview P2F | Transcript of Interview with Participant 2, female | 11/24/2010 | 65 min approx. |
| Interview P10F | Transcript of Interview with Participant 10, female | 11/26/2010 | 50 min approx. |
| Interview P15M | Transcript of Interview with Participant 15, male | 11/26/2010 | 45 min approx. |
| Interview P31F | Transcript of Interview with Participant 31, female | 11/26/2010 | 45 min approx. |
| Interview P36F | Transcript of Interview with Participant 36, female | 11/30/2010 | 45 min approx. |

| Abbreviation | Document cited | Participant Acronyms | Date | Duration |
|---|---|---|---|---|
| WS 1: P_ | Workshop No. 1 Transcript of final discussion | P1-P7 (P1-P4 female, P5-P7 male) | 10/28/2010 | 1:10 h approx. |
| WS 2: P_ | Workshop No. 2 Transcript of final discussion | P8-P15 (P8-P12 female, P13-P15 male) | 10/30/2010 | 1:15 h approx. |
| WS 3: P_ | Workshop No. 3 Transcript of final discussion | P16-P24 (P16-P22 female; P23-P24 male) | 11/04/2010 | 1:20 h approx. |
| WS 4: P_ | Workshop No. 4 Transcript of final discussion | P25-P32 (all female) | 11/05/2010 | 1:00 h approx. |
| WS 5: P_ | Workshop No. 5 Transcript of final discussion | P33-P39 (P33-P38 female; P39 male) | 11/06/2010 | 0:50 h approx. |

| Abbreviation | Document cited | Remarks |
|---|---|---|
| Quest. | Table of findings from the individual questionnaires (Workshops) | Clustered by questions and individual participants |
| Written statements | Students' poster documentation of small-group discussions and final discussions (Workshops) | Clustered by workshop and questions/discussion topics<br>Partly amended throughout the final discussions |
| Field diary | Field diary | Documentation of personal conversations, notes and field observations |

# *Annex*

*Annex Table 1. Students' Reflections on Migration*

| Group Affected | Positive Aspects | Negative Aspects |
|---|---|---|
| **Those who leave** | Gain international exposure, experience new life abroad, good life, experience other peoples' cultures, see beautiful places<br>Enjoy working with sufficient resources other than improvisations, have minimal workload outside<br>High chances to advance in education, in the professional life, school-wise, improving one's C.V.<br>Gain new knowledge and skills to apply in Malawi<br>Earn a lot more money than in Malawi, easy to develop yourself and your family after gaining money outside<br>Find good life partners<br>Come back changed, modernized, rich, look nice, attractive and very educated | Face insecurity because of racism, xenophobia, stigma and discrimination, problems in settling down in foreign land (>'stress induced psychosis')<br>Are regarded as people who do not love their country, cannot enjoy caring for people of our own nation, face acculturation > forgetting one's<br>Suffer from poor interaction with families and friends, break- ups, loneliness<br>Have problems to find good accommodation if you don't have relatives, problems to get medical services, problems with communication in terms of language, challenges with technology<br>Work with fear of being sued when a little mistake happens, can easily be sent back home<br>Have challenges to re-adapt to the Malawian working environment |

| Group Affected | Positive Aspects | Negative Aspects |
|---|---|---|
| **Those who stay behind** | Comfortable living in their home country | Suffer if those nurses who leave the country do not assist them financially |
| | Boost of economic status of the families and the community where migrants are coming from (money for school fees, good home, money to pay for better health services at private hospitals) | |
| **Nurses in Malawi** | Practice the ideal things which they learn in their setting | Wont get rich at all or maybe slowly |
| | Are close to their relatives, enjoy staying with their families, comfortable living in their home country | Suffer over-working, a lot of pressure is on remaining nurses in terms of workload, this reduces the quality of care rendered for clients |
| | Have better chances of attending workshops because some people are not available | |
| **Malawi in General** | | Malawi's government looses a lot of funds in training health personnel who leave without serving the country, waste of resources, the government will get poorer and poorer |
| | | Will face under-development of the country and increased mortality rates |
| | | Faces "brain drain" dynamics > motivation to migrate for the ones who stay, after seeing the good things that others bring from abroad |

*Annex Table 2. Core Nursing Cadres in Malawi*

| | |
|---|---|
| **Nursing Officers** | NOs are Registered Nurse/Midwifes (RNM) with a Bachelor's degree in Nursing and Certificate in Midwifery or RNM with 4 years experience at the next lower level respectively.<br>There is a hierarchy of grades from Chief NO down to Principal, Senior and simple NO.<br>NOs hold the highest rank among nurses and midwifes, assuming management and decision-making responsibilities and supervising NMTs. They are primarily located at district and central hospitals. NOs are critical to providing sophisticated nursing care, however are hardly found at health centers and hospitals in rural areas. |
| **Nurse Midwife Technicians** | NMTs are trained in a 3-years diploma programme. After 4 years of service they can be appointed to a Senior position of their cadre.<br>NMTs are mostly found in health centres and community hospitals, which often lack NOs. They are the mainstay of nursing and midwifery care in standard situations. |
| **Community Health Nurse** | CHN are only trained in small numbers, however they perform the important task of providing care in remote rural communities. They are trained in a 1-year upgrading programme. |

Sources: MoH 2010: n.p; MoH 2011: 9

## Perspectives on Development

edited by Petra Dannecker (Universität Wien) and Ulrike Schultz (Theologische Hochschule Friedensau)

Maria De Eguia Huerta
**How Can the Human Capability Approach Contribute to Gender Mainstreaming?**
A postdevelopment perspective on the dynamics of gender equality promotion in the international cooperation for development
vol. 1, 2017, 362 pp., 29,90 €, pb., ISBN 978-3-643-90782-0

## Social Protection in Health

Challenges, Needs and Solutions in International Health Care Financing
edited by Hans Jürgen Rösner

Gerald Leppert
**Social Risk Management Strategies and Health Risk Exposure**
Insights and Evidence from Ghana and Malawi
vol. 2, 2016, 324 pp., 34,90 €, pb., ISBN 978-3-643-90642-7

Hans Jürgen Rösner; Gerald Leppert; Philipp Degens; Lisa-Marie Ouedraogo (Eds.)
**Handbook of Micro Health Insurance in Africa**
vol. 1, 2012, 488 pp., 49,90 €, pb., ISBN 978-3-643-90171-2

## Studien zur Ethnopsychologie und Ethnopsychoanalyse

hrsg. von Werner Egli, Gerhard Kubik, Maya Nadig, Johannes Reichmayr und Vera Saller

Moya Aliya Malamusi
**Za UsingÆanga Ndi Ufiti – About Healing Practice and Witchcraft**
A Culture & Personality Study of Traditional Healers in Southern Malawi
vol. 9, 2016, 196 pp., 24,90 €, pb., ISBN 978-3-643-90764-6

## Defragmenting African Resource Management (DARMA)

edited by Dr. Mafaniso Hara (Institute for Poverty, Land and Agrarian Studies, University of the Western Cape) and Prof. Dr. Tobias Haller (Universität Bern)

Steve Donda; Mafaniso Hara; Maxon Ngochera; Erling Berge (Eds.)
**Fragmentation of Resource Management on the South East Arm of Lake Malawi**
Dynamics around Fisheries
vol. 3, 2014, 192 pp., 29,90 €, pb., ISBN 978-3-643-90505-5

Peter Mvula; Meya Kalindekafe; Paul Kishindo; Erling Berge; Friday Njaya (Eds.)
**Towards Defragmenting the Management System of Lake Chilwa Basin, Malawi**
vol. 1, 2014, 144 pp., 29,90 €, pb., ISBN 978-3-643-90398-3